HANG IN THERE

HANG IN THERE

Being the true history of how a healthy, energetic man was brought to the edge of death by a savage disease; of how he was treated with a protracted, controversial therapy; and of how he was restored to health more vigorous than that when he was stricken.

by DALE ARMSTRONG

Grossman Publishers ‑ New York ‑ 1974

Grateful acknowledgment is made to the *New England Journal of Medicine* for permission to quote from "Benefit from Alternate-day Prednisone in Myasthenia Gravis" by Dr. W. King Engel and Dr. John R. Warmolts (January 6, 1972).

In grateful thanks to every
one of the many who helped
to make the miracle . . . and
especially to Doris.

HANG IN THERE

CHAPTER 1

◆§ Nature, time and patience are the three
great physicians.—Book of Proverbs

In a private ambulance, bucking traffic from Connecticut to Maryland on a raw March day, an old man was being kept alive by a mechanical respirator.

He couldn't swallow. He couldn't speak. He had double vision and the lids of both eyes drooped, the left almost to closing. Arms and legs were abnormally weak. Hearing was restricted by the pressure of fluid in his inner ear. His mouth sagged, giving his face an apathetic, expressionless appearance. And he had not been able to breathe for the past fifteen days. When his intercostal muscles failed, he'd been hooked into an artificial respirator and, at the same time, since the swallowing muscles also were paralyzed, a nasogastric tube had been shoved through his nose, down his gullet, and into his stomach for food and medication.

The muffled sound of wind and traffic, the presence of the nurse beside him (ear tuned to the respirator's rhythm), the knowledge that his wife was riding in the chilly cab with driver and striker, that he was bound for a new adventure—all this did almost nothing to dissipate the sick man's feeling that he was alone, completely cut off from the world.

He was seriously ill with myasthenia gravis, contracted who knows when. Probably in the autumn of 1968. It was now March, 1971. He was on his way to the National Institutes of

Health in Maryland, just outside Washington, to play guinea pig in a research project involving his mysterious disease.

What had brought him to this pass? How had such an agile, active man, vigorous and replete with animal energy, been so sapped of his vital juices?

He had never before been seriously ill in his life, barring the week he was in bed during the influenza epidemic of the First World War.

When he was growing up down South, in Mobile, he was not what could be called a robust child. "He's peaked," said one of his aunts, who made two syllables of the word and sniffed disapprovingly at her sister's rearing of the young. It was true that he was thin and spindly, but it wasn't a sickly body. There was energy in it. Frequently he was fresh and flippant in a desperate effort to mask distrusts and inner tremblings. He did not very much like the people part of his world. He would retreat to the chinaberry tree that was hardest to climb, watch the June bugs dine in the neighboring fig, and try unsuccessfully to make some sense out of the tangled way in which his elders seemed to want him to behave. They had very strange requirements at times. He got along best with his grandfather's black help. Repeatedly he would risk the application of his grandfather's heavy leather slipper to his tender bottom by running away from the comfortable bed on Dauphin Street to sleep the fitful night on the porch of a shanty, where he felt he was wanted—though it was not wise to welcome him—and where he invariably wet his pants at first light. The return home, sometimes in convoy, was uncomfortable.

He was elementally schooled at Springhill College, an all-purpose school just outside the city limits managed by the Jesuits, which later allowed his claim that he had gone to college before finishing grammar school. There were two uneventful scholastic years in Salt Lake City before the family migrated to California, where he entered Hollywood High School and studied at Loyola College. He was an erratic student.

With his formal schooling at an end he went job-hunting. The only consideration was a pay packet, and so he was chivvied into ridiculous situations. For what but an envelope of coins does one want to wrap packages in an Irish linen shop? Or count bits of paper dealing with spark-plug sales and enter a number on a large sheet in a cramped hand? Or serve as office boy to a grubby little man who smelled bad through his eau de cologne and wore pince-nez from which a dirty, dove-gray ribbon dangled, and who peddled cemetery lots?

One day, when chance had hardly time to form itself, It came along. He recognized It at once. It was just what he wanted, despite parental warnings. He latched on to It with zeal and vigor, became a cub reporter and followed his father, long since an expert political journalist, onto the *Los Angeles Times*.

In the sea-kissed, milk-and-honey land that lay south of the Tehachapis and east to the Colorado River, there was no more vociferous voice than that of Harry Chandler's daily journal. Mr. Hearst's *Examiner* was a noisy echo, but it was the *Times* that had the class and the prestige. Besides, the Chandlers were rumored to hold mortgages on much of Mr. Hearst's Mexican acreage, the result of sneaky didos at a time when the Senator's son had indulged in unbackstopped overextension. Whatever the truth of it, a cachet of raw power was added to that of rank, and this all rubbed off agreeably on those who labored in the editorial warrens of the *Times* at First and Broadway.

The young man made the most of these benefits, far less through wile than happenstance and a mildly acquisitive nature that was quick to embrace opportunities. His daily and Sunday columns in the *Times* were powerful tools. They gave him entry into every corner of the fabulous world of Hollywood at its most glamorous.

In addition to this power of the press the loosely supervised columnist enjoyed, he used his strong and resonant voice to broadcast the news three times a day over the newspaper's radio station, housed literally in The Tower of the Times, a landmark, a crenelated finger that poked itself into the cerulean sky.

It was from this aerie that he began arranging commentaries and interviews with the medium's brightest stars and personalities. His roster was impressive: Jack Benny and Bob Hope, Lum and Abner, Amos and Andy, Fibber McGee and Molly, Fred Allen and Portland Hoffa.

After a while his own name got around, especially when he added movie-star interviews to his other broadcasts. And as the name grew, so did the income. Even sweeter, the vanity butter.

The inevitable sequitur to this frenetic activity was work in front of the motion-picture camera. Two of his casting-director pals, at Paramount and RKO, called him for work in half a dozen films. They were only small parts, until the Paramount musi-

3

cal in which he played the young millionaire, gussied out in tails, who gave the lavish costume ball for Ida Lupino—who was in love with Richard Arlen and not with him—and with Jack Benny and Ben Blue on hand to wassail it up.

He was paid exorbitantly.

For reasons now unremembered he never used that supple springboard to test the waters of the balmy pool. He was living in little more than twenty-four-hour segments. What's with ahead-planning when it is a lovely candy store where all the trays are free? And it would always be. There is never a depression if you have a good job and are eating on the uptown side of the porker. So he behaved as he felt like behaving, checked only by his own inner rules. There was more thinking with loins than head, and humors were being distilled in a soup of genes and chromosomes or whatever they were that neither of his immediate forebears would have recognized in a million years.

The times were such that while it wasn't entirely sensible to conjure everything in blacks and whites, it was far from a cerebral world. It was a time when it was easy to pick out people as oranges are culled. Some on this pile for juice, some over there for marmalade, some on this little pile for fancy eating.

He began seriously to look at people with an eye to discovering the treasure. Not old buddy-buddy, wrapped and ready to go. The woods were full of those. But somebody whose chemistry meshed and who, after a while, would still be comfortable to be with. And after a few more whiles hadn't said the wrong things and with whom there was no call to sham or dissemble. His quest was not an expedition to tear the Holy Land out of the infidel grip, but it was a search nonetheless. He was so eager to find the Grail that he tended to believe that much of what was said was so. It was not always so. Mostly not so. Rugs were pulled out from under him by these friends of short standing. And as time went by they would drop by the way. Good riddance. And the gamble was far from a costly one. To come upon what time would prove to be a true friend was such a bankbreaker it immensely outweighed the acrid disappointments that were, by the nature of man, high in the majority. In his life he had been a very lucky man. He had found nearly as many true friends as there were fingers on his hand.

Those sensual and exciting days seemed to be well marked by a tale his father used to tell about the spirit and the style of a

California that was gone but which, in a subtle way, and paradoxically, existed in parts of the still golden land.

He would roll the story off his tongue many times in the years to come about those early days when there were less people and more open land and the freeways were still dusty roads.

It was the custom then to provide food and shelter to whatever traveler came to the hacienda gate. When the meal was finished and the mount bedded down, the wayfarer would go to the room where he was to spend the night and there, on chest or table, would be a bowl of gold coins. He was welcome to take what he wanted or required. Quite often the bowl was untouched. It was a matter of honor.

Did such things mark those times as hospitable and trustful to a now-lost degree? Was this only a sentimental legend? No matter. True or not, the tale fit the land as neatly as the colorful boxes of a Chinese puzzle snuggle contentedly into themselves. The Sierra was a warm, snow-capped wall against too much reality. The sun did more than shine on this Eden. It grinned. Enormously satisfied with itself, that fiery star spent long, pellucid hours peopling orange groves with little suns, staining strong and virile bodies brown as berries and making it inexpensive to shoot Westerns in Griffith Park without resort to artificial light.

The young man lived all out in this emotional extravagance. Full speed. Head on. Work or play. What were to some long-hour labors were welcome to him, even when they were not all that rewarding. An agile, imaginative mind and a sense of humor, deportment of provincial manners and a deal of charm were able to move him, after a time, into those envied circles to which he possessed no ticket of family, money, or unusual talent.

Among his other chores he thumped the tub for such fabled creatures as Marlene Dietrich, Doug Fairbanks Junior, Basil Rathbone, Carole Lombard and Loretta Young. He worked for Howard Hughes on *The Outlaw*, getting considerable attention for the bebosomed one-time chiropodist's assistant who starred in the film with Walter Huston and Thomas Mitchell.

There were other oysters in this stew. One film with Eric von Stroheim and two with John Barrymore, with whom he shared an office on the balcony of the Warner Brothers colonial pile on Sunset Boulevard, finding that extraordinaire's interest in Bacardi and monologous conversation extremely heady fare. And he spent dutiful time with the "outlets" to gain favorable mention of his clients, Louella and Hedda being the glass rubies in the idol's eyes.

That was long ago and far away and there were two sides to the well-worn road. There were sins to think upon. These reflections seemed to come sharpest on the raw days of early winter in the East, when he had taken so many alien chemicals into his body that he was brittle as an autumn leaf, balanced precariously on the thin edge of a crisis.

Once again, not yet fifteen, he was in the orange grove in Alhambra, in back of his uncle's house, when he saw the bird in the tree. It regarded him with innocence as he slowly raised the air rifle and aimed it carefully at the beryl vest. Why? Need for a target? No fallen fruit, no empty can, no bottle in all the land? Why at that moment, when his finger began to tense, did not an ear-shattering and mind-exploding roar come rolling out of the sky or at least a cry from his own throat to send that animal to another and less violent death?

Nothing stayed his hand. He pulled the trigger. The bird fell dead. He stared at the small blue ball, among the rotting fruit, as if he had just come upon the scene, then turned and went away. It would make him miserable the rest of his life at the senselessness of that waste. What really pulled that trigger?

In the speeding ambulance, not yet to Baltimore, he thought a lot about his past—about the excitement of riding the firebreaks of the Hollywood hills in an English saddle, about a yawl across the channel from San Pedro to Santa Catalina Island. And how he'd had enough success in the business world to take him to London and Paris and Bombay and to an Arabian Nights date grove outside the capital city of Bahrein for a night of feasting and the gift of raw pearls from the ruling sheikh.

Alive. Strong. Avid just to be. Curious about the world. Moving with energy. So what was he doing here, flaked out in a jostling bed, too worn to be afraid? He could not pull a puff of air into his lungs or push it out again as other people can do so easily. And with a goddamned eyelid that wouldn't stay up!

That had been the first symptom of the disease that was upon him. Two and a half years ago.

In October of 1968, playing pool at his club, he became acutely aware of his inability to keep his left eye open or to hold his head up as he bent over the table, sighting along his cue.

Something was wrong. Probably one of those transient visitations that would go as it had come, as so many others had done. So he let it slide for another week. He never did like running to the doctor with every ache and pain. But when the weakened eye muscles persisted and the lid drooped lower and when his arms and neck began to follow, he became seriously concerned.

His internist in Greenwich, together with the community doctors he got in touch with, didn't know what the trouble was. They did check him into the hospital for tests, including brain scan and spinal tap, which was uncomfortable and scary. He didn't like it. When anybody shoves a long needle into the spinal canal, a number of unpleasant things can happen. It is a very sensitive theater.

Since the symptoms of his disease were common to other nerve-muscle problems, a neurologist was called in to consult. It was more than just a bit of luck for the sick man that Dr. Walter Camp had served at the National Institutes of Health and was uncommonly familiar with the sick man's ailment. He immediately suspected myasthenia gravis. Tensilon, endrophonium chloride, was injected intravenously, and the diagnosis was confirmed.

Tensilon, which dramatically restores muscle strength in one or two minutes, persists for only two or three more, then falls off, leaving the muscles as weak as before, clearly demonstrating whether the disease is present.

Thus, in February of 1969, five months after the lowering eyelid—a dangerously long delay—the man's affliction was officially entered into the record.

Myasthenia gravis.

CHAPTER 2

⋟ Dig! Dig! The jewel is hidden low.—Act of the Votaries

THE sick man had never heard of that disease before the doctors told him what was wrong. In the months to come he became intimately acquainted with it.

As he told those concerned enough to ask what ailed him, myasthenia gravis represents a breakdown in communications. The brain sends a message through a healthy nerve to a healthy muscle but at the point where they meet—the synapse—the message fails to get through or, at best, reaches the muscle weakly.

This debility, this syndrome of fatigue and exhaustion of the voluntary nervous system, is marked by progressive paralysis. And when the intercostal muscles and diaphragm fail, there is no breathing except by artificial means. Such failure can cause inflammation of the lungs and pneumonitis, and can result in death. Only a few years ago the mortality rate was as high as four out of five afflicted. Today the figure is reversed.

The chronic, noncommunicable disease, capricious as a zephyr, is aggravated by stress, particularly when pressures are prolonged, and by those drugs that increase the activity of bodily functions. Myasthenia gravis isn't generally believed to be an inherited disorder, although studies have shown that it occurs in families marked with the affliction more often than can be explained by chance. Genetics cannot be entirely ruled out.

9

MG, as the ailment is referred to in alphabetic shorthand, most frequently affects the muscles of the eyes, lips, face, tongue, throat, and neck, and then the chest and limbs, but not those of the heart, the bladder, or the intestines.

The cause of myasthenia continues to elude the best medico-scientific minds. There seems to be general agreement that the trouble exists in the nerve-muscle junction, where normal impulses pass from the neurons to muscle fibers by means of acetylcholine, the chemical that stimulates the muscle to contract.

The cause may be the failure to manufacture enough of this chemical or to permit its free release at the nerve ending, or it may be that there is some kind of inhibiting substance in the blood stream. Again, it may be that MG is an auto-immune disease, in which circulating muscle proteins, or antibodies, stirring up mischief—directly or not—interfere with normal muscle contraction.

There are other hypotheses. Research is under way to determine, if it can, the role played by the thymus, a glandular organ that sits on top of the heart and usually atrophies with age. The function of the thymus is uncertainly known, some regarding it as being concerned with early growth of the body and others believing it is involved in blood formation. In any case, experts frequently recommend its removal from the myasthenic. Always when a tumor is suspected or detected.

The first defense against the ravages of the disease is drugs. Their effects are not always predictable. What works happily for one patient can utterly fail another. Myasthenia comes rightly by its teeter-totter, unprognostic reputation.

Few of the muscles of the man in the ambulance had responded to prescribed medication with certainty or consistency. He had stumbled through a thicket of drugs, dosages, and time schedules in what turned out to be a futile effort to find more than temporary relief.

The mainstay of his intake was Mestinon, the trade name of the drug whose medical name is pyridostigmine bromide. It is the most popular of the drugs that are antagonistic to anticholinesterase, the enzyme that normally destroys acetylcholine, the chemical vital to normal neuromuscular communications.

Over the distance, he had taken as little as 24 and as much as 2,000 milligrams of Mestinon a day. A massive dose. At one period, he went from 50 to 750 to 80 milligrams a day in less than four weeks. That wasn't a tame roller coaster, either.

More than Mestinon had gone into his body. They'd tried Prostigmine, another anticholinesterase. It backfired. Aldactone didn't do any good. And he didn't have much luck with abenomium bromide, which has the trade name Mytelase.

He did some lucky-star thanking that he had escaped the more severe side effects of this chemical catalogue, although he was no stranger to abdominal cramps, nausea, diarrhea, profuse perspiration, excessive salivation, and urinary frequency and urgency, an uncomfortable and at times embarrassing condition.

There had been days of jitters and shakes, uneasy sleep turned into insomnia, and urination slowed to the point of pain, with ephedrine sulphate.

Atropine usually counteracts many disagreeable side effects, including reduction of excessive secretions that build up in the mouth and throat. But atropine can be a lethal danger by disguising the cholinergic crisis.

"Antidotes are poison," as Mr. Shakespeare said.

The gut absorption of these drugs into the blood stream is a highly inefficient process. By mouth, sixty milligrams of Mestinon puts less of the drug into the blood than a few milligrams injected into the veins. As the drug is broken down by the body's action, some goes to the liver, some to the synapse, where it is wanted, but the largest part of it leaves town by normal eliminatory procedures.

From this, it should be apparent why intravenous injections of potent drugs should not be done by amateurs. A slight measuring error can raise merry hell. Anticholinesterase drugs can loosen the bowels, which speeds the medication through the absorptive system and puts less of the drug into those places where it might do some good. *Ergo*, patient, disregard the classic physician's admonition. Do not try to heal thyself. At least, not with a hypodermic needle.

In the autumn and winter of 1969, the man's symptoms flopped all over the place, varying in nature and intensity not only from day to day but from hour to hour. The neck muscles would be too weak to hold his head up, his eyelids would droop, sometimes to closing, there would be double vision, swallowing muscles would fail, and his arms would go so weak he couldn't shave himself or brush his teeth. It was rare that he was ever free of one or another of these torments.

When the neck muscles went on strike, he was forced to hold his head up with hand under chin, sometimes for several hours. Except when he was walking or at table, it wasn't too difficult to make this prop unobtrusive.

At times, without warning, there would be a convention of symptoms severe enough to qualify as a minor crisis. On one occasion, after a day or two of reasonable calm, he found himself unable to swallow his own juices. They were filling his mouth and oozing into the windpipe, gagging him almost to vomit. And in mid-Manhattan.

He leaned against the corner of the Roosevelt Hotel, on Madison Avenue, as his breath began to come short and vertical double vision assailed his eyes. Which of his fellow pedestrians were flesh and blood and which were ghosts? Was the taxi hurtling toward him as he crossed the street steel or specter? He could not close one eye to shut out two of everything. Truly, he was a long way from home. Holding one hand under his chin and supporting himself with the other, he made his way slowly to Grand Central, waited nearly an hour for the next train to Old Greenwich, inwardly scared damned near to death that his folly could cost him so dear. What an unmitigated dumb, to get caught in midtown New York without any protection whatever. He didn't make that mistake again. From then on he carried the necessary medication wherever he went.

The sight of his wife, Doris, in the blue Barracuda, when finally the commuter clatter-box limped into the Old Greenwich station, was tonic. It was only a short mile up the road to prove the truth of the cliché. There's no place like it.

In those uncertain days, depending on the whims of his disease, home was a combination of heaven and purgatory, with the celestial side odds on. When the bad days would come along and he'd be so weak he was kept to his bed, his wife would look after him and make him comfortable and bring his meals. And the cats would come in and play fanciful games and explore the tops of the bookshelves as if they'd never seen any of it before.

SuSu, the seal-point Siamese with the vastly loving heart, was always the first to give up the chase-me's and gambadoes to come onto the bed and settle beside him.

Gimma, the finely marked Abyssinian, was pushing nineteen years, but this did little to suppress his feral nature or his keen sense of humor. As he joined SuSu he made a perfunctory pass at the page the master had just finished reading, with one eye covered because of the double vision, then found a select spot at the foot and settled.

Tiddles, the white alley-cat kitten they sometimes referred to as a "domestic short-hair," had been rescued on a back-country road from an oncoming truck whose horn he did not hear. He had been born stone-deaf. Joining the others, Tiddles would make as many as half a dozen tight turns before he curled himself against the blanketed leg.

These three seemed to sense the level of the sick man's spirit as they kept him purring company. It was very comforting.

On the better days he would do odd jobs around the house, fuss with gardening a little, rest on the patio, and if it wasn't a double-vision day, he might drive into Greenwich, five miles to the west, to do some errands. Or, if a Tensilon test had been scheduled, he'd report to the doctor at the hospital's outpatient clinic.

His sleeping, erratic at best those days, would be jolted at four in the morning by the travel alarm. Mestinon had to be taken every four hours around the clock. When swallowing was too unreliable to take the tablets, he had to pour the cherry-flavored chemical, a vile-tasting brew, down his throat with a prayer that gravity would do its stuff and none of the acrid syrup would be sucked into his lungs. His luck held.

Later, when his throat could handle solids reasonably well, he would take Mestinon "Timespan" tablets, each containing 180 milligrams of the drug, half of which was released during the first four hours, the other half during the next four hours. These extended duty tablets would control the symptoms until the morning dose was due, letting him get a full night's sleep.

Throughout all this medication mishmash—different drugs, altered schedules, fluctuating dosages—there seemed to be an almost aimless groping. On everybody's part. It troubled him. The doctors, some of them at least, surely ought to know more about the disease than they seemed to know. He had never regarded these practitioners as any more than ordinary people who had acquired varying degrees of knowledge of a particular discipline. Certainly they were not sensibly to be seen as demi-gods. And they were more than likely doing the best they could.

But the best that fails to cut the mustard is very much a feeble. What is wanted at such times is more certainty. Wider knowledge. Deeper insight. Better guessing, even. Not just "Let's try this and see what happens." That's blood brother to the old aviation jape: When the newly designed aircraft spins in on its maiden voyage, the designers give it a shrugging "Oops! Back to the drawing board" routine. Chilly comfort for the pilot.

If Mestinon wasn't going to do the job properly, what else did the pharmacopoeia hold? About the only drugs that they hadn't yet got round to trying on him were urocholine and anti-lymphocyte globulin (ALG). Urocholine had been used for some urinary problems and had been tried on a few myasthenics. Results had been inconclusive. As for ALG, it was alleged to cost $500 a shot and the side effects were supposed to chop up the white corpuscles, good and bad. It is an immunosuppressive, as opposed to the anticholinesterases. Bad lymphocytes, thought to exist in myasthenia, are only one expression of an immunological system gone haywire. Another: abnormal antibodies against muscle, found in one myasthenic out of three and in nine out of ten of those who had developed thymic tumors. Whether the lymphocytes or the antibodies or sickly humors from the thymus cause the weakness in myasthenia, who can say?

The sick man's less than meager knowledge of his affliction persuaded him that the world of medicine is long and flat, and if one isn't an able navigator, one can sail to the very edge of it and sometimes fall out of the world. Some do.

CHAPTER 3

The age of miracles is forever here.—Thomas Carlyle

To this day no one knows what brought on that dramatic event in October of 1969.

He was home in Old Greenwich. The day, like its immediate predecessors, had turned out to be singularly unsatisfactory. A sharp headache woke him ahead of the alarm and his depressive mood was deepened when he spilled his morning medication all over the desk, bathing in the viscous liquid a new book, a finished letter not yet in its envelope, and some miscellaneous papers. *Quelle* mess. The myasthenia bore on him heaviest when his defenses were dragging.

This was the day all pencils fell out of the hand. The furniture wouldn't stay out of his way. No glass of anything was safe from spillage. Long before drink time—what an Olympian concoction a Scotch-and-soda is—he was prodding the nest in his stomach where the worry vultures keep house.

The evening dragged dully, but he stayed up late, hoping to tire himself. No go. He still had a bad night. Next morning, with the sun streaming into the room, he made a startling discovery. His myasthenia was one with Nineveh and Tyre!

Somewhere in the dark hours of the early morning his disease had become no more. It had vanished.

Much obliged and *deo gratias*. He was cured!

No eyelid droop. No inhibited swallowing. No Jello in the

knees when he went up and down stairs. No clambering of any kind any more.

The meals were paradise. He ate and drank as normally as he had ever done. His voice was clear and resonant. If that wasn't cure, it would indeed do until cure came along.

This delightful normal human-being condition prevailed for nearly two months. He couldn't have been clam-happier. His doctor was pleased, too, and told him that spontaneous remissions from myasthenia do occur now and then—as had just been demonstrated—but that they were far from common.

"We haven't the foggiest idea what brings them on," he said. And added, cryptically, "They have to come before the disease kills you."

He never did find out what the doctor meant.

At the end of the seventh week, he fell off the horse. At three in the afternoon. The left eyelid went to half-mast. The head began to sag as he was driving a nail. He missed it completely. Throat muscles began to walk away from their chores and double vision again distorted the world. What the hell was going on?

He reached for the phone and called the doctor.

"We'd better run some tests. Can you come to the clinic right away?"

He got into his car and onto the road, wadding Kleenex under the left lens of his eyeglasses to thwart the heavy double vision. (He didn't learn about plastic corrective prisms until, many months later, his diplopia had been long gone.) He alternated the other hand between supporting his chin and hitting the horn in an effort to wake up the clods who seemed unaware he was having trouble with his driving. Double vision and head sag are not the safest seatmates when you pilot a Barracuda on a busy highway.

Never mind. He was sure that if he took it easy, held the head erect and kept one eye covered, he wasn't likely to run into anybody and nobody was likely to run into him. On this trip, at any rate, that's the way it worked out.

At the clinic he was started back on Mestinon. His myasthenia had returned, all right. In force. And now it was to be his closest companion, in varying degrees of intensity, until the autumn of 1971—that magic mark on the calendar when this

16

crippling, unpredictable, up-and-down, no rhyme-or-reason affliction would be contained.

Now that his daily living pattern was on "tilt" once again, he was sharply aware of the special inadequacies of his body. The throat and its environs were a major if not the main arena. What did he know about it, except that it let him breathe (though few people think about that until a stumbling block appears) and is the canal down which food and drink are sluiced.

The starting point, in this fascinating country, is the mouth, an orifice that is opened much more than necessary. It is also that grotto into which one can deposit the most succulent foods, to be bathed on their way with degustable wine.

Once inside this fleshy cavern, the potables and viands start on a short, dramatic journey to the stomach by way of the pharynx, the deeper part of the mouth, and the esophagus, the nine-inch tube that extends downward into the catch-all. On their way, they skirt the opening of the larynx, the voice box, to the lower border of the cricoid cartilage, which lies just below the Adam's apple. Medical types call it the thyroid cartilage.

The trachea, the windpipe, is another cartilaginous tube some four inches long and an inch in diameter. It extends down the front of the neck and then bifurcates (a fancy way of saying it forms an inverted vee) into the bronchi, which lead to smaller and smaller tubes in the lungs.

At the upper end of the trachea the larynx opens into the pharynx. The trick is get the larynx closed off during swallowing so that the epiglottis gets into the act and something they tell the medical students are the aryteno-epiglottic folds come front and center to shut off the windpipe opening. It's a neat trick but all most people need to be concerned about is that the epiglottis should remember what it is supposed to do and when to do it. And then does it.

A dozen different sets of muscles operate the vocal cords, which, when they are functioning, help prevent foodstuffs from getting into the trachea instead of into that Lucullan well, the belly. When the symphony of muscle machinery is out of tune, as in myasthenia, one can suck food down what used to be called the Sunday throat. This is what is meant by aspiration—globs of foreign matter pulled into the air tubes. All manner of problems can and do flow from this malfunction, including terminal pneumonia.

Until he'd done this bit of physiological homework, he'd thought the main function of the vocal cords was to produce song and speech. Live and learn.

Many times during his illness, the myasthenic pressed for death's sweet twin and was refused. How is the night to be passed when sleep is so elusive? There isn't even "ol'-rockin'-chair's-got-me, cane-bah-mah-side" to help the insomniac through the dark and sluggish hours. When you got the wakes, honey-chile, 'less you git he'p, you jes' aint goin' *no*-wheah!

It was pretty corny dialect but the sick man felt that once in a while, for apparent unconcern's sake, he had to ham it up.

The witching hour of the waking night would have spent it-self, with sleep as far away as ever. Dick Cavett had shut up shop. The Late Late, being almost more painful than Morpheus's absence, had been given the go-by. On almost all of these plasters that the cyclops regurgitated, the aging hero easily dodges the falling timbers in the bombed basement, zigs his way around naked switchblades, zags deftly out of the way of bullets from the gunsels who never seem to be able to shoot for sour owl-dung, and cleverly exposes the uppity lawyer for the cad he is, thus reaffirming that mother, mince pie, and the flag are the undying verities. Woe is me.

By now, the sick man's eyes had gone too red-rimmed for reading, so he turned to that otic triumph of the Golden Age, "the raddio," as Al Smith used to call it. There is a deal of magic in a 2½ x 4½ x 1½-inch black plastic box, with a little wheel for finding the stations and another little wheel for making them loud or soft or gone.

Settling back in bed, he plugged in the earphones. The night-talkers were on. Mostly pedestrian yammerers, as people usually are when they are too conscious of trying to cover too much ground too expertly. Surprising how few speak well in public.

After a while there came the point when the owl-gabbers lost the battle they always lose to someone. Even an insomniac can take only so much logorrhea. He turned the little wheel to silence. It was time for a more serious try for sleep, that most desirable of the three natural anesthetics. Fainting, apart from being out of fashion, is not the most satisfactory way to depart the day's cares and is usually more difficult to persuade than slumber. As for death—forfend.

Sleep is the tidiest option and when it is seriously stalked, the first step is to eschew unimaginative approaches. Sheep-counting and its cousins aren't worth a stiver. When he set his mind to it, having done it on occasion, the little death was not too difficult to come by. What had to be done was to latch on to a containable idea and squeeze it firmly. Something like space-gazing or beach-lolling or chess. Space-gazing is a deceptively simple form, requiring a purity of purpose and pursuit not everyone can summon up at will. Beach-lolling, which has merit in those areas where there aren't too many people and the water's not too disgustingly filthy, can hardly be classed as a manic activity, though at some of the southern strands there are likely to be erogenous diversions. A chess game is probably best. The Icelandic championships took it out of the ivory tower.

So settle for chess and in a quiet, dozy way, narrow the mind just enough to exclude the immediate world. Don't push too hard. Let the mind float, bringing it back to the chessboard whenever it starts to meander. And it will. Become concerned to the exclusion of everything else with the threat imposed when the rook goes to king five. Or see ahead to the disaster that's promised if the knight's poisonous fork is overlooked. And every time the mind strays, call it back, gently. With tenderness. First thing you know—dreamland.

CHAPTER 4

These are the times that try men's souls.—*Thomas Paine*

THE myasthenic's disease fluctuated wildly in the early weeks of 1970. He was closer to fragility than he or his doctors realized. Drug intake had been inched upward whenever the muscles faded, and by the end of January he was on the edge of a major crisis.

There are two kinds peculiar to his malady. The more prevalent, produced by underdose or the refractive unruliness of such drugs as Mestinon, is the myasthenic crisis. Here, the muscles that keep body fluids out of the lungs and draw air into them, make eating and swallowing possible, become too weak to do their job. The result is asphyxiation, aspiration of liquids into the lungs, pneumonia.

The other is the cholinergic crisis, the direct opposite of her deadly sister. Even trained medical practitioners do not easily diagnose this one correctly. The crisis results from an overdose of the very drugs that stimulate the muscles when properly administered. Treatment for either crisis must be given immediately. Misstep or misjudgment can tip the life-death balance.

Tensilon can perform a signal service at these crucial times. This potent chemical is used to test myasthenics, checking the adequacy of their dosage of Mestinon and similar drugs. If the dosage is adequate, Tensilon will produce a sharp but transient increase in strength. But if the patient has been overloaded, muscle weakness is rapidly intensified. Even the test has its dangers. Tensilon might improve some of the more obvious muscles and worsen such critical ones as those used in breathing. If not caught in time, it could kill.

Despite the signposts, not enough is known about these drugs. Patterns are difficult to establish. What is barely enough for one patient pushes another into a taut and brittle state. And they can produce an acute asthmatic attack, through contraction of the involuntary tracheal and bronchial muscles. This could well be what triggered his first bronchial spasm. He was walking through Grand Central Station on the way to a business meeting. For no apparent reason and without a scintilla of warning, the throat muscles began to twitch and contract, throttling his breathing. He was literally staggered as the airflow was sharply reduced and he realized that the simple, easy, taken-for-granted act of pulling air into the lungs was being interrupted to the point where he was going to choke to death.

Gasping, he made his way to the cab rank in Forty-second Street. Passersby stared at him and hurried on. He wheezed directions to his doctor's office uptown in a raucous caw that would have panicked Leonidas. The cab jerked into the traffic stream.

It turned out to be the granddaddy of all the wild-eyed, horn-open, never-mind-tomorrow cab rides Manhattan had ever seen. Spurred by the gaspings for air from the back seat, the bug-eyed cabbie cut around traffic against the grain, ran red lights, bulled two blocks contracurrent down a one-way street to reach the building on Eighty-ninth just off Fifth Avenue.

There was not much time to spare. The bases of the passenger's fingernails were beginning to turn blue. Not enough oxygen was getting to the lungs. He was no longer able to use the strictured muscles at all. His throat was almost completely closed. How much longer did he have?

The cabbie slammed his hack to a jolting halt, paused only long enough to lob an obscenity at the horn-blowing driver whose passage was blocked, and supported the stricken man into the foyer, where nurse and doctor, alerted by the doorman, took over.

The adrenalin injection quickly relaxed the throat muscles. Beautiful, wonderful, marvelous air rushed into the starved lungs. Crisis over. Welcome relaxation. Only problem now: did that prince of jehus get a big enough tip? The doctor's veteran assistant had known exactly what to do. It is always a pleasure to do business with professionals.

"Stay relaxed," the doctor said, writing a prescription. "Take this ephedrine three times a day. Let me know tomorrow how you feel."

In the waiting room the rescued man thumbed the magazines for half an hour or so, took a taxi back to Grand Central, caught a commuter train to Old Greenwich. Forgot all about the business appointment until the next day. He went to bed early that night. In the morning he didn't feel as bad as he thought he would. By the middle of the week the spasm panic had been pushed onto a back burner and he was caught up again in details of his newly established public relations consultancy. It held fair promise locally, and when the opportunity to acquire overseas clients came smiling down the pike, it looked like the lilacs were blooming in spite of his malady. So he booked a seat for his first flight in that hotel on wings, Boeing's 747.

His wife was very dubious about the trip. The doctors, she told him, should have advised against his going. Especially in light of the recent drastic spasm incident.

Time was to prove her out.

CHAPTER 5

~§ *It is the unexpected that always happens.—English proverb*

It was a sunny March morning when he arrived at Heathrow. Customs was easy. His clumsy, cavernous B4 bag wasn't all that heavy and in an hour he was installed in the Savile Club, on Brook Street, between Claridge's and Grosvenor Square.

The next two days were filled with business demands, errands, and look-arounds. He loved walking in the West End. On the third day he was taking a quick, light lunch at the Corner House, near Marble Arch, when, in the middle of a bite, he felt the throat muscles begin to twitch and grab. He had barely time to wash down the half-masticated lump of food before the rasping began and he was fighting for air.

It was New York all over again.

The young couple across from him, startled into staring, were inactive for no more than a moment. Properly they placed knife and fork onto plate as the now-wheezing man fumbled his doctor's card out of his wallet and showed it to them. At once they took over in that competent, quiet manner that makes even a tinge of flap, let alone alarm, utterly unthinkable.

Collecting hats and coats, they supported the seriously stricken man to the street, hailed a taxi, and took him to Harley Street. Almost before they'd passed Portman Square he was sucking less and less air into his lungs. He had checked in, on his first day in London, with Dr. Raymond Greene, world-renowned for his expertise in treating myasthenia. It was the best insurance the choking man had ever laid in.

That taxi trip was forever. Not nearly the verve of the Manhattan cab ride. By the time they had turned into Harley Street, he was a fish out of water. The doctor's needle stemmed the spasm and loosened the constricted throat, just as had been done on his Manhattan go-round.

Again in control of himself though still a bit weak and apprehensive, he settled the tabs for lunch and the taxi, gratefully thanking the young man and his wife for their help. At Dr. Greene's suggestion, he agreed to go next day to New End Hospital for X-rays.

When they were ready for examination, the films seemed to show the presence of a thymoma, a tumor, on the thymus gland. It wasn't a certainty. The X-rays weren't all that sharp. A more precise report was wanted. Dr. Greene arranged for a session of thymic venography with the man who had pioneered this special technique.

The venography had been set for the following Tuesday at the Royal Free Hospital in Gray's Inn Road. It proved to be an interesting exercise. It was neither comfortable nor comforting.

The building in which the Royal Free was housed was as old as any ghost-ridden castle in the British Isles. And there were so many twists and turnings on the way to the X-ray area that it seemed to be a good idea to scatter bread crumbs to help find the way to the street again when the myasthenic had been thoroughly explored.

Checking in at the proper section, he was relieved to note how bright and efficient the nurses were. Pretty, too. And despite the architectural antiquity of the high-ceilinged rooms, there was a general air of no-nonsense, heads-up business about the place. While he was no expert on the subject, it seemed to him that the radiographic equipment was as modern as any he had seen stateside.

The doctor who was to perform the venography was short, dark, intense, and articulate. The myasthenic was ably briefed, gowned, and tabled. A heavy camera was pressed down onto his chest. Left arm was extended over the small table that supported gauze pads, tape, and a number of small instruments. Seating himself in front of the fluoroscopic screen, which rose behind the table, the doctor fiddled with control knobs and a small, sharp, impatient knife.

Incision was made elbow-high. Supine on the table, the victim was able to twist his head just enough to see the ghostly picture on the small screen as the catheter was inserted and pushed, twisting and turning, through the veins that led circuitously into the thoracic cavity.

Periodic introduction of an iodinated, X-ray-opaque substance marked the way toward the thymus gland where, if there was a tumor, it would be found. But after nearly half an hour of backing and filling this venographic excursion had to be abandoned. The catheter's progress had been stopped by a too abrupt turning in one of the veins and could be persuaded to go no farther.

Another vein was located, a new incision made, and the flexible tube reinserted. Nearly an hour later this trip had proved no more successful than the first and the exercise had to be regretfully concluded. The doctor muttered his dark displeasure at the failure and apologized to the patient for any discomfort in a way that plainly told he knew whose fault it was.

The myasthenic had long since had enough of this intimate invasion of his body. He was glad it was over. His arm was tender for a week. And whether a thymoma was lurking in his chest had not been settled. He was troubled and disappointed at this loose end but there wasn't anything he could do about it, so he walked slowly back to the club on Brook Street, hungry and tiring more rapidly now than even a few days back, wanting only to get down a glass of warm milk and crawl into bed.

He was more than miserable, huddling in that chilly, alien room. The promised business was out the window. He was in no condition to meet prospective clients, let alone persuade them he could solve some of their problems. There'd be no opening of a London office this trip. If ever there was to be. And he was far too rocky to pull much pleasure out of his favorite city. He was anxious to get back to more familiar territory to cope with his malady.

By this time he had taken such a quantity of drugs that his muscles were losing their ability to respond. His body was becoming insensitive to medication. Refractory. Brittle as glass. The current dosage, on top of the medicine that had already been poured into him, was no longer containing the disease. Symptoms were increasing in severity.

The sick man had stayed on in London only a few more days. He was taking Mestinon every two hours, for a total approaching two thousand milligrams a day. He was rarely free of cramps. His bowels were loose and the sphincter grimly unreliable. Nausea would strike at odd times, working with his weakened muscles to keep all but liquid food away from him. He was down to less than ten stone. One hundred thirty pounds. He had lost fifty in less than a month.

The day before his last visit to Dr. Greene, who was to tell him he was sure a tumor was present and that it had better come out, one of the grimmest episodes of his illness occurred.

He had just left The Running Footman, where he'd been able to manage no more than half a bowl of soup and some milk to flush down the Mestinon tablets. Down Berkeley Street and along Piccadilly, he headed for Leicester Square where, out of sentiment, he hoped to find the fancy billiard parlor he'd visited when he first came to London years before.

As he walked down Coventry Street he knew he'd never make it to the square, less than a block away. With no more than this faint warning, the urge to defecate pressed heavy on him. In panic, he realized he had completely lost control. Sharp pains wracked him as he tried desperately to get across the street and into the public convenience. He didn't make it. The physical problem was bad enough; the psychic shock was brutal.

He duck-waddled the rest of the way, crawled down the twenty steps, found a tanner in his change pocket, popped it into the slot, and entered the pay toilet. Shaking with rage, he did what had to be done, tried to clean himself with handkerchief and the tails he sawed off his shirt with a penknife, and disposed of his shorts. He climbed to the street again and hailed a cab. His anger and confusion were larded with fear that the disease and its drugs were growing to the point where he might be unable to cope with the demands of his body. It was a stupid, dismal, messy state into which he had fallen.

The final visit to Harley Street was to talk about the suspected tumor and how best to get rid of it. Dr. Greene described in detail how the thymectomy would be handled, if it was decided to do the surgery in London. It struck the sick man that cutting through the breastbone to get at the malignant sweetmeat was dangerous surgery at best, and especially so for a man as old as he was. The doctor agreed. It might be well, he had suggested, to consider radiotherapy. Perhaps it would be better all round if he got on an airplane and went home. His doctors there might have some ideas about prolonged X-ray treatment, although as it turned out, they didn't give it much elbowroom. How effective such treatment might have been in his case, he would never know. Neither would the doctors.

On the TWA 747 out of London airport, almost before they'd cleared Land's End, the throat muscles began to tighten, just as they'd done in the Corner House a month before, and in Manhattan before that. Cold creeps began to dance in his stomach. It wasn't easy to talk himself into sitting back quietly to draw slowly on the bronchial inhalator Dr. Greene had given him against just such an emergency. The air passages were slow in opening and he was ready to go into the bag at his feet, pull out the needle, and give himself a shot of Tensilon. Before he could locate the ampule the muscles unlocked, air stumbled down the windpipe and then flowed evenly once more. The big problem the rest of the trip was trying to make sense out of the adult movie. But it was some time before the sweat had dried and the acid smell of fear had gone away.

When he reported this spasmic incident to Dr. Camp on his return to Connecticut, he was told in brisk language how dangerous it was even to think of using Tensilon on himself. His abysmal ignorance of his complex disease and of the drugs associated with it could easily have proved fatal. Minute measurement mishaps could put too much or too little of the chemical into his system, bringing on a crisis. Besides, it was adrenalin, not Tensilon, that was needed to stem the spasm. Tensilon could very well have been the poleax that would send him angelward.

An airplane over the Atlantic at thirty thousand feet is not an ideal place to cope successfully with that kind of gymkhana.

CHAPTER 6

No doctor at all is better than three.—German proverb

THAT April he was busier than a bird dog.

The myasthenic was checked into a New York hospital for ten days while the respiratory experts tried to find an answer to the breathing problem. They didn't.

The X-rays they'd taken in London had been sent on by airmail days before. After more than a week they still hadn't turned up. His doctors ordered tomographs redone in an effort to locate that thymoma. In this sixes-and-sevens situation, the sick man began to think seriously about Dr. Greene's suggestion of radiation therapy. Maybe he ought to go back to London for the treatment and if thymectomy appeared to be indicated, have it done there, sternum split to the contrary notwithstanding. Certainly it would cost a packet less than the medical charges that would be run up in New York. And maybe the London mediciners knew more about myasthenia gravis than anybody else. They were the pioneers in this neuromuscular morbus, weren't they?

The invalid was flailing about in the snare the ill are so often caught up in when they are not being treated successfully. Get away from wherever you are. Go somewhere else. Try something new. In a way, it isn't as silly a system as appears at first blush. The more rides on the merry-go-round the better the chances of hooking the brass ring.

Before anybody else could get around to being serious about the notion, the sick man nose-dived spectacularly and had to be whisked into hospital again. They set up the operating room.

Dr. Alan Kark was to be the surgeon. He was a blond South African. Did fine work, the patient was told. It turned out to be quite true, but the thought did strike him that it wasn't likely he'd hear from one staff member that a confrere was less than an able plumber. As this cynical thought crossed his mind, the myasthenic berated himself. He was getting mighty picky, which is just a few doors away from bitchiness.

Day and time were set. Dr. Kark came in late in the afternoon for the presurgery talk. He set the sick man at his ease at once. Choosing his words carefully, the doctor spoke precisely, in a gentle manner. His accent was twin brother to Basil Rathbone's splendid voice, as he explained what would be involved in the surgery. He had decided not to cut through the breastbone. That further endeared him to the queasy man. Instead, Dr. Kark would make a transcervical incision above the sternum and go down into the thorax in front of the lungs to snip the offending organ away from its anchors.

The majority of surgeons like to lay the chest open and have a good look round to be sure they've made a clean sweep. Those in the South African's camp regarded the transcervical technique as easier on the patient and, if they have to, can go in again to pick up any of the gland they may have missed. The best technique? It's still a debate. The effects of thymectomy are far from determined.

In a hospital study of 270 of these operations, 240 were sternum splits; 30 were transcervicals. Myasthenia was severe in the large majority of the cases at the time of surgery. Some of both sexes benefited but the results varied. Thirty-five percent achieved remission within several weeks to several months after thymectomy; others responded after an interval of several years. In a few, myasthenia developed after surgery, clearly indicating that the thymus gland is not always essential to occurrence of the disease. In addition to the remissions, 41 percent improved, 7 percent remained unchanged, 2 percent got worse, and 15 percent died.

The Connecticut myasthenic hadn't fallen into the latter category by the time they wheeled him out of the recovery room and into ICU (Intensive Care Unit), and it was too early to tell about the others. They did say he'd set some kind of a record, being the oldest patient to undergo that kind of surgery. It was a wry claim. Not much to preen on. Didn't make him feel a bit better when he heard it.

Almost as soon as they'd moved him into ICU they began making him ready for his first course of ACTH (adrenocorticotrophic hormone). Initial stage was cold turkey. Complete and immediate withdrawal of all medication. This was more than a disagreeable exercise. Cold turkey had sent some myasthenics into total incapacity, it was that rough. Happily, he hadn't been marked for this kind of dramatic emergency, although as the drugs faded out of his system little worms began to crawl around inside him and make his skin itch and his muscles weakened almost to immobility. It took nearly four highly uncomfortable days for him to lie there, like a blob, on the edge of being too impotent to be apprehensive.

The mechanical respirator was breathing for him through the hole in his throat. Tracheostomy had been performed when they took the thymus out. He was not comfortable connected to the crate-like breathing-machine. There was difficulty in establishing an easy rhythm. The inspirations would come too fast or too slow. The air intake seemed inadequate. Not enough air would be a common complaint all the time he was in ICU. They were stingy with air. Maybe they figured it would stretch the stricken muscles into greater effort. They may well have been right. But to the sick man, they were oxygen misers.

And there seemed to be a lot of fiddling with the respirator's switches and buttons, checking dial readings, calculating oxygen flow and huddling in little, smocked groups whispering professorially and writing calculations onto charts.

Early on the tenth day, the patient began to have trouble with his eyes. There was intermittent diplopia. But seeing double didn't matter much in that sterile room. The trouble was he couldn't close his eyes properly, and hearing was increasingly muffled. Pressures had been built up in his inner ear by the respirator. Almost all outside sound had been shut off. He was in such a misty state that he didn't care much what was going on around him until the sharp pain bit into his shoulder.

Something was pressing into his flesh. He tried to lift himself off whatever it was. No go. When the nurses came alongside his soggy bed, he tried to make them understand something was wrong. No go. He couldn't tell them what the trouble was. When the cuff of the tracheostomy-tube is inflated, all air is cut off from the voice box. The full flow from the respirator goes directly into the lungs. There'd be no scribbled note. He couldn't hold a pencil. Finger muscles were on strike. Shrugs and grimaces were unintelligible. It was a hell of a time to be playing charades, anyway.

The pain increased. A hemostat had been left in the bed, after his last tube-feeding, and somehow had worked itself under his left shoulder, digging into his body.

All afternoon went by before it came time to turn him on his side to change his breathing posture. The stray tool was discovered. It took quite a while for the hurt to go away. What bothered him most—he was feeling pretty sorry for himself—was that instead of some kind of sympathetic concern for the accident and his discomfort, there was a distinctly whoopsy-daisy attitude at the misadventure. In his mind he turned the nurses into callous witches. However they might be at any other time or place, in ICU they were not for him. Cross-examine him and he'd swear they went about their work as if they liked everything except the patients. Some people sure need a passle of hand-holding.

The myasthenic decided early that the nurses reflected the character of the man in charge of the ward, an Englishman with a hyphenated name, which didn't endear him to his critic. This piddly prejudice must have been an outcropping from his provincial past. He realized that bias against a name that's parted in the middle wasn't very grown-up. But almost everybody has moments of small-mindedness.

The British doctor didn't seem to the sick man to be as interested in his patients as people so much as adjuncts to his machines. When he looked at the myasthenic it was as if he were not there as a person. It was like a mechanic might regard an ailing motor that needed a valve job. There seemed to be a good deal of laughing it up with the nurses, too, which bothered him considerably.

The chemical conflict between doctor and patient graduated into open hostility the day the Englishman strode over to the sick man's bed as if he'd been caught lighting a cigarette in a room where oxygen was in use.

Apparently he'd be using the call bell too frequently. Split-name bawled him out. Too much calling for the nurses, he said. The sick man had been having a particularly uncomfortable time and he wanted attention. So he'd pressed the button too often. So what the hell? He was damned glad he had enough strength to shove the button deep enough into its shallow socket to light the overhead beacon. He wanted them to make him rest easier. The doctor didn't see it that way.

Strong, healthy, good-looking (but not as handsome as he fancied himself), he stood beside the sickbed and said in a cold voice dripping with accent butter, "You will simply have to stop pressing that button so much, you know. You are ackshally becoming a nudge. We haven't room for nudges, you know."

Nudge, with that speech, became an unfriendly word. No longer a gentle push. No more a reminding jog. Use and inflection had made it an insult.

"If we have any more trouble," the healer of the sick continued, "we'll have to send you down to General Care."

That wasn't the happiest of prospects, so he kept his finger off that call-bell button. Unless it was something as acceptably important as a bedpan, he cowed himself into enduring discomfort, which churned the frustration acids in his stomach.

The four-bedded rooms on the General Care floors could be more depressing than ICU. When he had been installed on the third floor he almost wished he were back upstairs in ICU. The man across from him was dying with afflictions that gave him no peace. Day and night they sucked blood out of a hole in his side, as fresh bottles of blood and plasma were hung on the IV (intravenous) tree. His piteous moans were punctured by wailing cries of agony at all hours. And in reedy whimpers he would call out for his mother, the appeal to the last refuge.

The bed on his right held a man of sixty or so who went hot and cold with metronomic regularity. Day and night, electric blankets had to be piled onto his chattering body. Minutes later, mattresses of ice. In addition to these frenzied afflictions he couldn't or wouldn't control his bowels. Cleanup and linen-change made that bed a very active area. Each bed-change time, the dusky, dumpy nurse scolded the man for failing to call for the bedpan. He never responded, which raised the level of her complaints. In the quiet hours, they would disturb what little sleep went on in that room.

The man in the third bed was quiet most of the day, staring at the ceiling. It was in the early morning hours that he would hammer on the guard rails with whatever came to hand, making the metal rods clang to the accompaniment of a singsong crying out in a strange tongue. Deprived of any instrument, when the monkey was on his back he would beat on the rails with his fists. On two occasions they had to strap him into restraint until his convulsion had spent itself.

Several times during these dramatic incidents the room provided every day, there would be delays before necessary nursing care was applied. The more critical demands, where even a slight delay could bring on serious consequences, seemed to be met immediately. But in the lesser matters, they were devil-may-care. It seemed to the myasthenic that the nurses, or many of them, were cavalier about their jobs, working as waiters in cheap restaurants work. Doing no more than had to be done, giving only what had to be given, and that almost grudgingly.

When two of the nurses, who knew each other well, were sharing four patients they were out of the room for long periods. Coffee breaks and bullshit sessions went undisturbed by the myasthenic's call bell, which was tied to his left wrist so that if it fell away from his hand he could retrieve it and wouldn't be without some means of summoning help. Irony in a lacy costume. If he did use the little bell in a crisis and nobody answered, what good would it be? What would happen? He'd probably turn into a terminal statistic. It was a chilly thought. Suppose his fluids built up to the choking point and he couldn't call for suctioning? What if the Bird respirator faltered or conked out and air was cut off from his lungs? Respirators, like a lot of other machines, are not infallible. What if? Indeed, what if.

Tinkle, tinkle, little bell. Hope to be heard. Hope very much to be heard—and heeded—when the sick man is squeezed in a tight, frightened sandwich of fear and pain. And there is some nagging anxiety in that sandwich, too, with frustrations perhaps the largest slabs.

How could he make it known how terrible he felt except to be able to tell how terrible he felt? There was regularly now the familiar tightening of repeated hamperings, the rope's fibers singing in rising pitch. He would try to hold himself in, taut and rigid, clearly aware that as he did so he was barring the door to escape for the devils that were tormenting him. The point would then be reached when it was no use to fumble any further for relief or even for changes in the pressures. And all because of a silly, antic, childish thing. The little tinkly bell at his wrist.

His feeble, spastic fingers could not adjust it as he wanted it. He couldn't tie the white tapes tight enough to hold it in a place where it would not be too difficult to ring to summon help. Given time—and he had plenty of it—he would have made it. But the nurse, turning from whatever she was doing, brushed his hand away, with some impatience, as with a child, to set the cord *her* way. Say she was trying to help. This simply wasn't the way to go about it, damn her stupid soul. He shook his head at her and tried to reach the tapes again. She brushed his hand away again. The pressures rose rapidly. It was as if a thick oak door was weighted on his chest and faceless figures came out of the darkness, one by one, to lay heavy stones on the wooden slab and fade back into the misty nothingness.

How many stones? How many straws? How many drops of water? This is the kind of time that is not measured by the clock. Look, this is a ridiculous thing. How can a pudgy, unattractively uniformed woman, now small-minded to vindictiveness, lead him into such feckless, juvenile combat? For Christ's sweet sake, this monumental confrontation concerns the adjustment of a bell cord around a scrawny wrist!

So intensely did he silently form the words that he was startled when they did not leap the barrier of his stricken throat and shout themselves aloud.

Abysmal woman, don't you understand that any old knot will not suffice? The bell must not be out of the zone my flabby muscles can cover. So let's tie the cord *my* way. No, bloody goddamn it—tie it *my* way. *My* goddamned way! Tie it so *I* will be able to reach it if I must. Get your hands away from there or I shall surely kill you. Why can't I speak now, of all times to need to speak, to make clear what this is all about, to blast a pinch of understanding into that cemented brain? Lady, listen to me. I skate on the thin ice of panic as I lie here, unless I am sure I can call for help. If you tie the cord that way, you silly, pot-head bitch, my fingers will not—do you hear me—will not bend enough to grasp the handle if I need to ring the fucking bell!

This professional woman, who was not behaving professionally because of some pressures she was not able to withstand that day, was wrestling with the wrong adversary, behaving as if the only solution was control. She was wrong on many counts. And did she think the conflict had been concluded? That the duel had decided the issue? Did she think she was dealing with a rational being at that time and in that place? The body conflict was over. The clash of wills went on in force. As she turned away from the bed her very posture, innocent at other times, was the trigger and the firing pin and the ultimate straw, all rolled into one.

He called in all the strength he could muster into the wasted arm and struck out blindly, catching the near corner of the table by the bed, sending not nearly enough noisy objects tumbling to the tiled floor.

Startled by the clatter, the nurse stiffened into that cliché posture of exasperation. It was insufferable. He glared at her with hate of rare purity. The blow had been aimed at her, and reaching its mark would have relieved the pressure that brings small boys to strike show-off poses and run and yell in an effort to explode the compelling charge. Like Hitler at Compiègne, jigging. Like the man in the sweaty bed sending bottles and cups onto a noisy, unyielding floor.

The cursing had erupted in his head with the impulse to throw out his arm. He knew instantly how inadequate it was, yet he made no effort to stop the flood of the phrases. Summoned were goddamns and sons-of-bitches and bastards and puking pricks, amid the frantic, fruitless search for more potent expletives—deistic, scatological, forbidden in any fearful way. Fury added to frustrated fury at the lack of the savage sound of the human voice in anger. There is only one way to curse so that it has meaning. Strong and blasphemous words must be strung together with imagination and delivered in a roaring bellow. And here there was no sound at all.

As fast as it had come upon the stricken man, the shabby incident ceased to matter. He and whatever reservoir had been filled to overflowing were drained. The incident was over for now. But it would rise repeatedly from this burial to prod him with the prongs of contrition.

CHAPTER 7

It never rains but it pours.—English proverb

IT was that Intensive Care Unit again. This time it was unexpected eye trouble in addition to ptosis and diplopia. What made it worse was that it could easily have been avoided.

The sick man was so flaked out he couldn't remember how many days he had been doing cold turkey. It was not long after the hemostat incident. For several days the burning sensation in his eyes, as he lay in the sodden bed, was increasing beyond discomfort. The problem wasn't getting through to the nurses, either. And the doctors were too busy playing with their machines and stopwatches and charts to take any notice. So nobody came round to have a look at his eyes or put anything into them to make them burn less. He had no choice but to suffer the stinging irritation and keep his finger off the call-bell button.

It was two days later, when he had been moved out of ICU into the General Care room that the eye specialist was called in for consultation. By then the eyes had become severely inflamed.

The little eye man was a diffident, gentle person with steel-rimmed spectacles, mildly unruly hair, and a bulbous nose with a dimple in the end of it. He looked like he knew more about bookkeeping than ophthalmology. Not so. He knew at once what the trouble was and set about dealing with it.

Because of the myasthenic's ptosis, which caused him to tilt his head back to see from under the marquee of the drooping lid, he could not completely open his eyes. He couldn't close them, either. Thus the not-quite-closed lids left part of the cornea without adequate protection. Tender membranes began to dry out. The itching, after a while, gave way to active pain.

In treating his eyes, the doctor blinded him completely, to give them rest and let the medication he squirted into them make its best effort. Gauze patches were placed over his eyes and sealed tight with collodion. For four days he was blind as the man brought down to Gaza. And when the patches were taken off, the cilia stuck to the gauze fibers and some of the fiery liquid that was softening the collodion bonds got into his eyes and burned brisker than the fires of Tophet.

The damage, as it turned out, was not permanent. The painful experience did reinforce his attitude toward the ICU doctor he held responsible for the neglect. More coal was heaped on this fire when, after he had left the hospital, he received a bill from the British practitioner for "services." Since the hospital charged $225 a day for ICU services, he didn't see what justified the Britisher's bill for $315.

Arrogance on top of greed, he called it.

Such practices can give a profession a dusty name. In the myasthenic's book there was another mark against medicine.

All in all, he'd had a hairy time in ICU. It was in this sweat-soaked bed, weak almost to dormance, that he thought he was going to die.

As if he had gone into a strange room for the first time, he sensed rather than heard the burbling sound of the respirator begin to fade away. There were people around him, but he couldn't see them, enveloped as they were in a darkening curtain that moved slowly toward him, tightening the small circle of light in which he lay. He was sure this was the end of the line. To his great surprise, he was aware that he was not afraid. He had always thought that when his time was up, fear would predominate. He did not want to go, in spite of how dreadful he felt, but there was no fear, none of the stomach panic that was supposed to grip most men at this passage in time.

Then, as people naturally accept the impossible in dreams, the sick man was no longer lying in bed but standing, as if he were about to acknowledge high audience acclaim, in the lighted spot that was now narrowing more rapidly. He was no longer conscious of the breathing-machine or of the tube in his throat or that he was at all ill-disposed. No sounds from beyond this dark wall came through to him. He felt himself move in an odd, undulating manner, as when one walks on a waterbed. The movement was sensually pleasant but aimless. And the entire world was gone. He was alone. Utterly alone. Suspended in nothingness.

Across his mind flashed unrelated scenes, as if a strip of film had been clipped and spliced at random. When he was conscious again, trying to reconstruct this strange event, he would be able to recall no more than a single frame in that remarkable kaleidoscope. Nor would he be able to find any language that would at all accurately tell what or how he felt during the indeterminate time the scene was played. He was simply there, sensing rather than seeing the narrow sidewalk alongside the house leading to the barnlike building it was imperative to reach.

For only an instant he had taken his eyes away from the walk, for he did not see the transformation. But when he looked again it was awash with a film of water. Tiny whirlpools ruffled the surface, giving unmistakable warning of great danger.

He accepted the diresome threat as quietly as if he had been offered a cup of tea. Quietly he rejected the danger and immediately, in direct contradiction, started to dash toward the building that was, at no surprise to him, slowly receding. Suddenly, in midstride, he froze, aware of a presence by the side of the walk which had now become a river, branching into a waterfall that was cascading in the same direction as the water flowed, in complete defiance of Mr. Newton's law but fully accepted as quite a natural thing under the circumstances.

As these bizarre affairs crowded in on him, he readily recognized their lethal threat. Yet, as if he had never attempted it, he made no move toward flight. And he wondered, as he looked around him, why there were none of the deviate, grotesque creatures of the kind that people the paintings of Hieronymus Bosch, which somehow belonged in the scene. He needed them there to tell him unmistakably that all this was fantasy.

The sensed presence, human and yet not human, that had been beside him from the beginning, was guiding the flow of the river and of the waterfall. He stood there, suspended and with no interest in what he was watching. Of a sudden, as if a deep-throated bell had been rung, waves of sound washed over him. He knew the time had come. In sighed relief he relaxed and lost consciousness. In that infinitesimal time between the onset of the fainting and its completion, which did not seem at all hurried, the man knew that the light would come on again.

He was back in his ICU bed, eyes closed, listening to the muffled sounds of the respirator and to the moving of the nurses in the ward, a way off. In an odd way, he was not the same man who had almost gone on the long journey. Not everything— perhaps not anything—would ever be what once it had been. Values would change. Judgments would alter. Once this close to death, very little remains the same. And it mattered not one whit whether he would actually have died. He was never sure whether it was then or later that he came to realize that all of the discomforts of his illness, in the many months he was to suffer them, would not be as difficult to withstand as if he had not had that time in the darkness. His spirit had been braced into a sturdier staff for the body to lean on over the rough spots. It had been a rare gift. A rare gain.

As the little blonde stretched to hook the plastic bag onto the IV tree and reached for the tube in his nose—it was feeding time—his inner smile broadened.

Alas, he said, how sad it is, but this is not a perfect world. Sometimes great losses go unrecorded. In the days to come, when he would take occasion to recount his near-passage, there could justly be regret that no memorable deathbed language had been heard. It wouldn't have had to be a master poet's classic phrase, but a little something would have been nice.

On occasion he had pondered on a more serious side. Complex questions were involved. Questions to which no answers have been found. Such as when do the dying relinquish the right to determine their remaining days?

Never, was the sick man's answer. Each human is entitled (by what power he never identified) to do what he wishes, if he can, with his life. How and when he dies, if that can be handled, is his right, too.

How sacred is human life? Under what conditions is it right to be sustained? And who shall define the conditions? How treat the mongoloid? On whose assent the final easing of deep pain? And how important is the life of an Assam peasant or a Zulu? And to whom? Slide down the scale in this soul-searching catechism and one has to ask about the lives of bald eagles, stray cats, and guppies. The honest answers are sometimes reluctant to be counted.

However his neighbor saw it, the myasthenic knew how he wanted his end to come. It would be great good fortune if, on his last day, he was fit enough to handle himself. And then to die in his sleep. That would be great good fortune, too. Failing that, he didn't want to be kept alive as a helpless hunk, having medical types exercise their skills to sustain vegetable breathing, while appalling monetary boulders were added to the already heavy burdens of protracted terminal illness. To use ingenious devices to prolong the lives of the helplessly, hopelessly ill is gross obscenity.

He had made it clear in his last will and testament that when his living was over he wanted his life to be stopped. There was a reciprocal pact with his wife and an understanding with his sister on this matter. Now, having taken this difficult step in firm resolve, he found himself deeply relieved. To relinquish or conquer anxiety about death is to make peace with oneself.

Where indeed does life begin and end?

By no means always at birth or death.

In the days that followed his adventure, when he thought about it, other complicated questions arose to flex their muscles.

How weak the reed that the meek shall inherit the earth? How close to what actually took place is preached today about a desert sermoner who promised to pave the way to paradise? Is it better to conform than rebel when the moral stomach turns? To shut-eye than to pry? To follow the more profitable pursuits?

Along with these massive conundrums we live in a clutter of little things it is difficult to play hookey from, too. Even when we do take time to struggle with them, there is rarely wisdom enough to begin untangling the complexities.

This evening, just before he said good night to the cosmos and set ear to pillow, he heard another question clearly: When is an illness so hopeless that the time has come to throttle life?

He did not search long for the answer he knew did not exist as blanket truth. For each man has his own response. And so, practically, the myasthenic turned his mind to a mate-in-two chess problem and was asleep in minutes.

CHAPTER 8

◄§ First psychiatrist: "Good morning."
Second psychiatrist: "I wonder what he meant by that."

His body now cleared of foreign drugs, the first ACTH needle went home in the right buttock.

ACTH is rugged therapy.

On each of ten successive days, one hundred milligrams of the chemical are injected into the gluteus maximus, that bane of the overweight, with sadistic delight in some cases, if one may judge by the forcible manner in which the little sword is scabbered in the flesh.

Almost invariably, by the third or fourth day thereafter, the ability to breathe diminishes sharply. Other muscles are progressively weakened and almost complete helplessness takes over around the halfway mark.

There may be subtle differences to the scientists but to the myasthenic the paralysis of cold turkey and that of ACTH at the bottom of the barrel are one and the same. His brain remained alert throughout the entire course. The brisk bee-buzzing in his ears was tidal in intensity. He would drift off at times, then surge in again on high-crested rollers, his senses sharpened by the ordeal.

He was on one of these peaks when the bluff, bebellied doctor came bedside on his morning call. The big man's gleeful chortle, as he saw with relish how weak his patient had become, triggered all the vexation the flaked-out blob could muster. He seethed at the doctor's delight.

"Aha," the ursine doctor would aha. "We're weak, are we? Good. Very good. That's what we like to see. The weaker the better."

It wasn't as sadistic as it sounded. It's an ACTH axiom that the weaker the patient during the course, the higher the benefits are likely to be.

As with other myasthenic matters, this axiom was not constant. Sometimes yes. Sometimes not so yes. No two myasthenics are alike. Before the sick man was out of the woods he would learn not to count on anything. Well, almost anything.

He was on the respirator now and too weak to do much of anything. And there were a thousand questions he wanted to ask. Might not have been given the answers even if he had his voice or was able to hold a pencil to scrawl his queries on a little pad. The big doctor was overcrowding his hours, as he habitually did, in his effort to cover the entire waterfront. He was always impatient for his next patient. Half an eye could see there was nothing more he could do at the sick man's bed. The drug was working. Nothing could speed or halter its action. Now it was time's turn. But the Connecticut myasthenic was looking out of another window. He wanted believable assurance that he'd make it. That wasn't in the cards. The doctor muttered another brace of "good" sounds and took his leave. He was off to repeat his "hurrah, you're weak" performance for other miserables laid low by ACTH.

The weakened man did not like his doctor very much right then. Didn't like anybody in his room, in the ward or the hospital or in as much of the world as anybody would care to include.

It wasn't that he saw the doctor as a monstrous lump of insensitivity so much as he felt there was a more sympathetic way to play the part. That borderline Santa Clausian ho-ho-ho business was strictly Hollywood. Either the doctor was laying it on with a trowel or he wasn't all that good an actor. It didn't occur to the sick man then that he was asking a lot more of his doctor than a competent medical discipline.

Days later, on the way out of the ACTH straightjacket, the myasthenic reflected on the encounter. It is clear truth that each of us can behave only according to our nature and our business.

The sick man's contact with many of his doctors and nurses on the ward was sometimes brusque and chilly enough to set up severe stomach storms. How much he himself contributed to this *démêlé* was probably not inconsequential. What matters where the fault be laid. There was conflict. In the healing business, it is the professional who's required to cut through most of the knots. To discover how best to provide psychic easement to the sick, in spite of how provocative they become. Not always an easy task, to be sure, pressures of time and disposition being what they often are. But the artist settles for no less than the best he can provide.

With myasthenia, especially, stress is not good therapy.

In May, on his way out of the ACTH slough, a tall and gangling man came to his bed. It was Ichabod Crane with an oily smile. A smile that turned on and off like a light bulb when he set his mouth to speak. As if he had been convinced that the proper thing was to smile but hadn't been told what a smile is actually for.

"I am Doctor Frebbelgrup," he smile-said. It sounded as if he had said Frebbelgrup. Then, more clearly, "I'd like to talk with you, if you don't mind."

The moue dabbled on his lips and instantly killed the encounter. The meeting was DOA. It would never last the journey now, no matter what the distance.

"How do you feel?"

The sick man didn't want to use the word, but "lousy" came to the head of the class.

"Do you know what day this is?"

He did. He said "Tuesday" with an exasperated expression of petulant disgust that anybody in his right mind would ask such a question.

"How much is six and nine?"

He nit-picked at the lapse in grammar with perverse satisfaction. It reflected on professional aptitude, old boy.

"I make it something like fifteen."

"Do you feel depressed?"

Come on, now. How does a man as sick as he was know if how he felt was depression or myasthenia? Poor appetite, which was next on the list, is one of depression's classic symptoms. So flip a coin. Depression or dormant muscles?

How about lack of sexual interest?

Lackaday. At his age and in his condition he wasn't likely to be on the torrid Priapean side. Only once in all his hospital time had he awakened to a creditable erection in bed with him. He wasn't able to do much about it at the time, being all that weak everywhere else, except to let it behave like the proverbial old soldier.

By now there was little further to go in this psychic Twenty Questions. As for other symptoms of depression or mental instability, the myasthenic reckoned his sleeping problem to be disease-connected abjection, apathy pulling an oar in the same boat; and his digestive trouble a not unnatural consequence of filling his innards with a verminous witches' brew. As for lack of energy—come *on!* He had a very tidy pile of lack of energy. His goddamned muscles wouldn't work.

Before twenty minutes had been rung up, the interview had fallen apart. What the shrink thought about his interlocutee was not revealed at that meeting, but it would have been an insensitive witness not to have a hint. By no means did the sick man see his mind as a problem. Of course, in fairness, one had to concede that most folks are far from free of one kind of hangup or another.

And that was that.

Except for the bill. Seventy-five dollars.

As the beneficial effects of the ACTH depressed his symptoms and he gained in strength, the afflicted man would wander out of his room and meet some of his neighbors. On one of these shuffling excursions he discovered the "ambu," that manually operated respirator that was to be his constant companion for many months to come.

A young black, myasthenic for five years, had been given a new ambu for his birthday. It seemed a bizarre gift for a lad who definitely didn't have everything. At any rate, that's what he got. Gift wrapped.

The bladder-like bag, about the size of a football, had a plastic nipple fitted to the hose that protruded from one end. In turn, the plastic tip fit snuggly into the opening of the tracheostomy-tube in the throat. Squeeze the ambu in normal breathing rhythm and air is forced in and out of the lungs.

So the Connecticut myasthenic bought the young man's old bag, which wasn't as cosmetic as the new black, shiny leather one but was still in excellent working shape. With an ambu, no myasthenic is ever going to expire for want of air. As he rolled this comforting thought around on his mental tongue he recalled the grim story of the myasthenic who became suddenly too weak to reach the medication on the night table and so was lost. Well, that kind of thing wasn't going to happen to him. His ambu was a gilt-edged insurance policy. Unless of course there was something in the diamond type about unless the arms are too weak to reach or the hands too paralyzed to squeeze.

Never mind such dire unlesses. The ambu *was* insurance. That rubber bag was indeed a life sustainer and for a long time he carried it wherever he went. And well he did. On more than one occasion he had cause to use it.

The ambu fit neatly into a Mark Cross leather carrying case that also held a spare trach-tube, a small bottle of Mestinon syrup, another of tablets and Timespans, atropine capsules, an ampule of Tensilon, and a hypodermic syringe, just in case. There were two disposable gavage bags (to hold the food formula when he had to feed himself away from home), several large syringes, and a roll of paper tape; gauze pads, dressings, tissues, swabs, and hydrogen peroxide for cleaning the stoma and the trach-tube in his throat at least twice a day.

In the early stages of his disease, following surgery and his first cold-turkey session, ACTH encompassed him to a degree that he could not do very much for himself. But when he'd climbed onto the up side and could manage it, he dealt ably with his daily care and sustenance. The leather carrying case gave yeoman service.

The first ACTH course, in May, 1970, was not what the myasthenic thought it was going to be. He was seriously disappointed that it was not literally a ten-day course. From into to out of, at best, was a harsh three weeks. And being told he would get very weak midway was considerably different from the actually getting weak. But at the end of those strung-out weeks of atonic helplessness, when the muscles had come alive again and some of his strength had returned, the rigors of the therapy were almost fully forgotten. For he saw this ACTH as a cure, surely. It was true that the doctor had never said so, but the patient was too high in commutation now to recall the omission. In time, he would come to reflect that doctors seem to have a paranoic avoidance of the word "cure." Especially in myasthenia.

On the morning of May 21, pleased with his progress, he was eager for the doctor to make his hospital call. He wanted to remind him that the swallowing muscles were working once more.

Not perfectly but strong enough to put down a glass of fruit juice and a soft-boiled egg without too much effort.

Bathed and shaved, he was standing at the foot of his bed when the ursine physician came into the room, ward doctors and nurses in tow. The patient's grin had a slight touch of *l'homme qui rit*, since the face muscles weren't doing their best, as he made it clear that he'd "swallowed more than a thousand cc. yesterday. You said that if I could swallow that much, you'd . . ."

"So you're feeling better, eh?" The doctor's smile was more evenly distributed than his patient's. "Sounds like you want the tube out, eh?"

Whereupon he leaned forward theatrically, grasped the gastric tube firmly and jerked it out in a single, sweeping gesture. A muffled squawk escaped the myasthenic as mucous adhesions in nose passages and gullet were ruptured. Tender tissues were exacerbated enough to complain for hours afterward.

The patient looked down at the foot-long blackened end of the tube, eyes stung to tearing, ignored the staff giggles and said something about going home.

"Tomorrow."

"Thanks, doctor. I'm very grateful."

In the morning the swallowing muscles were materially stronger. Stamina had begun to make itself felt. It was sensual to pull air so deep into his lungs. It didn't take him long to dress, pack, and leave the hospital. Stepping onto the pavement boosted his spirits as if he'd mainlined Benzedrine.

By the middle of July he'd been home for two weeks. There was a lot of sitting in the sun in the patio. It was a bonus day if the blue jays were dive-bombing the cats on the hill. He didn't do much gardening or puttering about the place. Too weak still. Tired too easily. Oddly enough, swallowing didn't seem to be as easy as when he'd left the hospital. He began to have to wash the food down with milk. There was no trouble taking the Mestinon syrup, although that medication wasn't exactly a gourmet delight and the odor was particularly offensive to Doris. The cats didn't like it, either.

Under her care he'd gained weight. Up nearly 15 pounds from the 125 he'd scaled in May. She'd insisted they give her a specially prescribed diet sheet before her husband left the hospital. She followed it religiously. Meant to see that he got his health back if she had anything to do with it. This British-born's sense of duty and obligation was almost formidable. He was lucky she was on his side.

Old routines began to take shape again. He pecked at the typewriter. Letters mostly. Read as much as he could, although sporadic diplopia showed up to trouble him. No single symptom he was experiencing was all that bad. They didn't persist for very long when they did occur. It was the swallowing difficulties that fretted him most.

Maybe the trouble was that he was sitting around doing very little but worry about himself. Maybe it was time to see if there was a world out there and, if it happened that there actually was, have a look at what it was doing.

So the very next day he drove to the station, Doris taking the car shopping from there, and found himself battling the New Haven's sick-unto-death's-door commuter train into Grand Central, faithful ambu bag in tow.

It was good to get back to the office. If he could just get himself stabilized, just find the right dosage pattern and stay as well as he was at that moment, he was sure he could manage to stay afloat and pump some blood back into his anemic business.

The hope was a weak reed.

In what turned out to be a few short weeks, eye and throat symptoms recurred increasingly, intensified, and were joined by others. His slide downhill was drastic.

Halfway to Grand Central, on a Thursday, he realized he had left the ambu bag at the office, was grabbed in the stomach-pit, and rushed back to get it. Made a later train than usual and had to take his medication en route. Went out onto the platform, the toilet cubicle being too foul to endure, to make it as unnoticeable as possible.

He was more than an hour late into Old Greenwich and when he failed to spot the blue Barracuda, he was punched in the gut again as he realized he had failed to call his wife and tell her he'd missed the agreed-on train. He phoned from the station. She came down to collect him, still suffering from the deep worry that had flooded her when he wasn't on the train she'd gone to meet.

Dinner was on the somber side that evening. The fire was warming. He loved the open fire. The cats were sweet company, as usual. But it wasn't a good evening. That night, looking down at his bed in a faint fog, he found himself repeating almost to the point of gibberish, "No. Oh no. No." He didn't want to accept what was so as so.

Almost before he could say "knife" he was back in the hospital in New York and a nurse was sticking a needle in his arse.

The second ACTH course (begun in the third week of June) was blood brother to the first. He was discharged, weighing 125 pounds (down 50 and kitten-weak) on July 10. There were a few weeks of remission and he was back on his back again. Two down and, though he didn't know it then, two to go.

With this tour going off the road after little more than three weeks, the pattern of that unpredictable disease began to get more predictable. ACTH was rugged and costly. Benefits, though very welcome, were fleeting. For what he got out of it, after those severe bodily and psychic buffetings, it just didn't seem like a sensible way to run a railroad. He almost chuckled at the phrase as it formed in his mind. Considering the unspeakable New Haven, the comparison was almost ridiculous.

Before that week was out he had fluctuated in both strength and stamina, each valley a little lower than its predecessor. It was abundantly clear that this kind of charade was far from good enough to live with. If he had to spend the rest of his life in and out of hospital three or four times a year, with oppressive drain on body, spirit, and purse, to hell with it. Such a modus vivendi was uncomfortably close to vegetable living, larded with the frightening prospect that he might go downhill to little more than a blob, lying there with his world no more than stuff being put into him and stuff being taken out of him. And thinking. Even the faintest whisper of thinking would be dreadful.

This grisly notion fretted him more than it should have. He would wake up in the night, on occasion, with the fingers of fear in his gut. This wasn't like him. He had never been a frightened person. Rarely borrowed anxieties from the what might happen. But he wasn't the same now, and this changeover troubled him. While he still had control over his body, he told himself, he had to find an acceptable way to go through the gate before he vapored off into immobility.

It never became clear in his mind how he was going to make this passage. He didn't approach it as an immediate problem, the self-destruct theme being one he was characteristically disinclined toward. Better let it simmer until he got closer to decision time before seriously moving in on the problem.

Next morning there were more practical concerns, such as trach-tube care, coping with excessive secretions, making diary entries, and calling Dr. Camp to talk about drug-dose adjustments.

Just before lunch there was a dramatic moment when Gimma, the feral Abyssinian, brought a bird to him as a gift. When he took it from the obviously proud cat he discovered that it was alive and unhurt. He thanked his little friend profusely, opened his hand, and watched the bird fly high into the oak on the hill. The cat regarded him as daft. Whatever was wrong with humans that made them not so very bright at times?

One night during the third week in August he was awakened by a dream of frustration. He would set out to catch the very important train but was always diverted by one thing or other and so always missed it. This was a dream he had dreamed many times before. It had always been dismissed on waking. This time it had some measure of reality. It alarmed him somehow. He was worried, as he'd never been before, by the dream's outrage of reality that was this time no outrage. His body began to sweat. There were beads forming on his forehead as he leaned out of the bed to reach the lamp button. Breathing became difficult. Eyes filmed a little and double vision almost leaped on him. The sudden alarm bell startled him severely. It was time for the 4:00 A.M. dose of Mestinon.

With one eye on the measuring cup, he poured the ruby syrup and tossed it off. That was a mistake. The liquid started down his throat but failed to clear the opening into the windpipe. He aspirated. Severely.

The hacking, gobbing, wheezing rales brought his frightened wife into the room, fumbling with the clothes she was flinging on over her nightdress. She knew an emergency when she heard one.

They delayed only long enough to telephone the sleepy doctor, crawl into the car, and rush through quiet, rain-soaked streets to Stamford Hospital. In the emergency room they eased the spasms. Dr. Resnick arrived. A nasogastric tube was poked through his nose into his belly. And before the cock crowed he was bedded in the Intensive Care Unit. He'd added another hospital to his growing list.

The crisis had been successfully met and he was dozing. Doris had not yet been able to unwind and was far from dozing.

When her husband's strangled fight for air had twisted hard the knots in her stomach, they'd been pulled exceedingly tight by her fear for his life and by her helplessness to deal with the crisis.

"What can you do at such a time? When a child gets something in its throat and can't swallow, you can pick it up and gently pat it on the back. But you can't do that with a big man. You'd be surprised how big you are when I can't do anything for you."

His myasthenia was not his burden alone.

Next morning they readjusted his drug dosage. Symptoms subsided. After a while he went home. By now he was beginning to know a fair amount about his affliction and had developed a few shortcuts for coping with it. Some of the physical requirements became easier to handle with practice, although the self-nursing routine was always a nuisance. Sometimes it was even odious.

When secretions and viscous mucus began to build up heavily he rented a portable suction machine and set it up bedside. The sound of the tiny motor seemed just this side of a huge dynamo's shrill whine in his room. In the still of the night, when he had to bilge-bail himself, what must the neighbors have thought?

For all the fussy details of looking after himself, there were general rules it was sensible to follow, pegged to a theme with mild crusading overtones: Minimum physical effort. Maximum mental calm. More information.

If there was to be a way out—and he rarely believed there wasn't—it had to come through control and knowledge. So he strengthened his resolve and borrowed a book from his doctor. He didn't expect too much to come from this kind of medical inculcation, but it made sense for him to learn enough about his elephant so that he didn't have too grotesque a picture of the beast.

In the fabled days they told about the blind men who were bade to describe the rajah's prized pachyderm, an animal they had never seen or even heard about.

"It is the trunk of a giant tree," one said, running his hands up and down the beast's leg.

"Ah now," said another, feeling the tail. "It is a rope."

"A fan," pronounced the man at the ear.

"Not at all, brethren," came from him at the trunk. " 'Tis a snake. A huge snake."

"Naught but a rough and calloused wall," said the man thumping the massive body.

Each of the sightless witnesses was right enough and wrong enough to persuade the myasthenic that inconclusive bits and pieces of information are sometimes less valuable than no information at all. Better turn his natural inquisitiveness up a few notches. A little serious study couldn't hurt. He opened the book and began to read about the synthetic hormone that had demonstrated such strengths and weaknesses to him.

ACTH—adrenocorticotrophic hormone—is a pharmaceutical hormone of the anterior pituitary gland that stimulates the adrenal cortex, that firm, yellowish outer layer that makes up the larger part of the adrenal gland. This hormone urges the gland to produce its own natural hormones, which do a number of salutary things: crank up the body to respond to stress for hours and days, as adrenalin does for only a few short minutes, boost blood pressure, turn fats and proteins into dispersible energy, and spread anti-inflammatory substances throughout the body to fight various diseases.

Even the scientists who are well acquainted with ACTH, antibodies, hormones, and steroids, don't yet know how many substances other than steroids, if any at all, or even how many steroids, are released through the action of ACTH. Nor do they know whether ACTH affects more or fewer body systems than does prednisone, a similar chemical. Prednisone is a steroid that's used for a variety of therapeutic purposes, including successful suppression of the inflammatory aspects of such diseases as rheumatoid arthritis, nephrosis, and that terrible "butterfly rash" affliction, lupus erythematosis.

There is a considerable history of the use of ACTH in the treatment of myasthenia gravis. The National Institutes of Health, one of the nation's major facilities familiar with its use, administered three hundred ACTH courses to more than a hundred patients from 1966 to 1972. Mt. Sinai Hospital and Maimonides Medical Center, keeping joint records, administered some three hundred ACTH courses to more than one hundred patients from 1966 to 1972. More benefits than not were derived, despite a 5 percent mortality rate.

While it is true that a given ACTH course produces variable results, about three-quarters of those myasthenics given daily injections of one hundred milligrams of ACTH gel for ten consecutive days are reduced to helpless weakness after the first several days, which explains the glee exuded by the Connecticut myasthenic's doctor that made him want to spit into the Hippocratic eye.

There isn't much for it, when the body is squeezed into the slot right next to total immobility, except to indulge in such luxurious thoughts as puckering up a good, substanial expectoration. Or just to be able to spit, substantially or not. What bliss that ejective exercise can conjure up. Never mind the target. Into the wind. Through the fingers, to ward off the evil ones. Just to spit. Ah, joy.

Maybe the muscles will come round to it with the ACTH.

CHAPTER 9

It's a long road that has no turning.—English proverb

EARLY in their association, when his Greenwich doctor was having difficulty finding an acceptable pattern of medication for his patient, Dr. Kermit Osserman had been called in on consultation. This renowned physician was considered one of the most expert in the treatment of myasthenia gravis. His delivered opinion was that ACTH might set the sick man right, and so it was ordered. His was not a flat-out promise of recovery—but the halt are of a stamp. With greater clarity than that of their healthier brothers they hear what they want to hear. The sick man expanded the big doctor's prescription into solid prediction.

Thus, when the first courses brought no more than short-lived relief and the debilitating symptoms returned in force, the myasthenic was deeply disappointed. Morale flipped onto the down side and it was little comfort to hear the savants nod their heads together and speculate that short, intensive ACTH courses might well be the way to do the trick.

"Single weekly shots is the best therapy we've found to date," Dr. Osserman said on one occasion. "It doesn't always work, of course."

"We get good results with paired courses," he'd remarked at another time, with equal authority. "Benefits from paired courses last two to three times longer than from singles."

Paired courses of ACTH meant back-to-back treatments.

Three weeks of misery, a few days rest, and then another dive into the barrel. Such sessions are not a day at the races. A single ACTH course is a rugged, wrung-out, hairy sweat. Back-to-back has to be hell's delight.

The specialists in myasthenia have gone on record that "corticothropin is a poorly understood, empiric measure."

By the second week in September the sick man had so degenerated that another ACTH tour was inevitable. There wasn't any other therapy available. It was agreed he'd go through another course, but the sick man dug his heels in against returning to that hospital in Manhattan.

Apart from his aversions, he knew what it meant to his wife to have to make the rickety, thirty-five-mile commute to the 125th Street station, walk the less than safe and scenic sidewalks of that thoroughfare to Fifth Avenue, and take the bus down to 100th Street to visit him. She paid no attention whatever to his demand that she save her strength and give up the rigors of that long trek. And she wouldn't cut down on the number of days of call.

So he opted for Greenwich Hospital.

Dr. Camp demurred.

"Why can't we do it here?" the victim wanted to know.

"They've never done one here. They don't have any experience with it. I don't think they'll want to do it here."

The reluctance was understandable, even if it wasn't acceptable. When a myasthenic gets into the serious weaks, after three or four days of injections, it is a very good idea to have nurses on hand who know what the score is, who can detect the subtle sick sounds as readily as the more raucous sputterings, and who can cope with the emergencies because they have been down those streets before.

That's all very well, he made quite clear. The therapy will be done in Greenwich Hospital or no therapy.

So they undertook it.

It was the first such treatment administered in that hospital, where none of the ICU nurses had ever taken care of a myasthenic. Since he had undergone two ACTH courses it was only natural that he should don the expert's robe. Those who have survived grim experience tend to exaggerate its perils and to see themselves as the prime authorities on the subject. And so, propped in bed in the little care room that faced the nurses' station, he sounded off on the care and feeding of the myasthenic, giving the mildly amused girls pointers on suctioning and trach-care, and how to do a tube-feeding without spilling the goo all over the patient and the bed.

It was a novel classroom, that niche in the ICU ward. The pupils were delicious females. Some of them were pretty, all of them attractive. They were professionals with varying degrees of experience, and they knew a good deal more than they were letting on, just to please him. Chatter and natter as much as you will, invalid. It won't be long before the talk muscles fail and you won't be wording it up for quite a spell.

For a sickroom, it was a pleasant place. The patient was removed from the other beds by the partitions. There was a view of sky and trees, through which poked one of the ubiquitous white New England church spires. And there was an undercurrent of good spirits and humor that took nothing from the staff's serious concern for their responsibilities.

Sick as he was it warmed the cockles of his heart.

One day, when the ACTH courses were long gone and done with, he recollected that phrase and the occasion when it had come to his mind. What indeed, he asked himself, are the cockles of one's heart? Webster failed to tell him. Not even the Unabridged, which his sister had given him on his fifty-fourth birthday. All that this fascinating tome would say was that cockles are boats and ovens and shells but nothing that has to do with the human heart. Before having done with his incidental research, he wondered if it could be that the medics were following false trails for viruses, antibodies, and faulty electrical connections between nerves and muscles. Maybe after all there were Little Men, mysterious but potent invaders, who bring on myasthenia and who, among themselves, are known as Cockles and who make their home in the heart. But if this were so, as of course it could be, why would anybody want to warm them?

This pleasant flippancy aside, there was one thing he was sure of. Good nursing, as was evidenced during his third ACTH course in that fine community hospital, is more than bringing medicines on time or changing bed linen or rubbing aching backs or sucking the juices out of burbling windpipes. Much more indeed. It is also catering a birthday party for a sixty-eight-year-old myasthenic.

When his wife would visit him that September 28, she would bring along some funny birthday cards and some presents.

There'd be aftershave from the three cats, who were very clever at remembering anniversaries. And when he'd seen his gifts, Doris would take them home to wait for him. This time there'd be no candle-crested layer cake with gay, colored-icing inscriptions.

Even so, he was not to be entirely denied. As soon as the morning chores had been wrapped up there was a short, nurseless calm on the ward and then all but one of the six on the shift trooped into the tiny care room in a body, softly chanting the traditional natal hymn a bit out of synch. They bore, on a huge white tray, as if it were John the Baptist's head, a saucer of ice cream in which a tiny, lighted candle glittered gaily.

What a magnificent tableau. The floor doctor, passing, grinned from the door. Despite the tube impediments, the patient exploded into choking laugher that instantly upset the rhythm of the respirator. A few raucous gasps, a slight adjustment, and he was breathing regularly again. The inner glow of sheer delight was almost white hot.

By now the confection was melting enough to tip the taper into the cream to sputter out its flame. The party was over. Yet the love-warmth generated in that room by the simple scene coated the walls and filled the crevices. Some future resident of that room would one day feel its presence and be comforted.

On the fifth day of his Greenwich tour, early in the evening, his heart began to bounce around erratically. Something new had been added. What it meant the sick man didn't know. But it alarmed him. It startled and frightened him as if some idiot driver had come screaming around the corner against the light just as he was starting to cross. Here, on the flat of his back, how could he jump? What a time for another complication. A dumb, jerky heart. Balls on it! Nuts! What frustrating insanity it was to have to lie there with a mad glopping in his chest, wondering if maybe the sign-off button had finally been pushed.

The hurried signals located the doctor. He wasted no time sticking a needle into the patient's arm. The flutter subsided and disappeared. The sick man read the doctor's face as serious. They didn't talk about it. Too busy bringing in a small black box, a cardiac monitor, to set up on the window ledge.

When the wires had been connected, a thin, blue line jerked onto the screen from the left, made a bleep as it peaked sharply, straightened out, bleep-peaked again, repeating this performance until it went off, stage right, and a new set of blue-line bleep-peaks came on again on the left.

The invalid found it comforting to watch the machine, especially since he knew that it was hooked up to the nurse-station monitor. He was under surveillance every minute of the day and night.

It was better than television, that little box. And no commercials.

Lunch on the first day of October was especially delicious. He had been able to swallow it well enough to persuade his doctor that the irritating NG-tube ought to come out. The old throat muscles were in there pitching. It could turn out to be a no-hitter. So this time they snaked the tube out slowly. It tickled but it didn't burn the tender tissues. And the lower quarter of the plastic duct that had rested in his belly was as black as sin, just as the others before it had been. Somehow, he thought, black seems to be an unfitting color for the stomach. What's wrong with pink or ecru?

He went home the following Tuesday in better shape than the first two ACTH courses had provided. Maybe improved morale had something to do with it. And maybe the cumulative effect of the three therapies was beginning to pay off. He hoped so. It was just a thought, but he felt it didn't hurt to have hopes. Even if sometimes they did get chopped off at the knees.

Early in November he bundled up and went into Manhattan. It was good to see his pals at The Players. Out of the corner of his eye he caught a few somber head-shakes, inspired by his scrawny, less than robust appearance. He did indeed look a little like death warmed over. Didn't stay long at the club. Tired too easily. Cabbed back to Grand Central and caught an early train home. Not enough meat on the old bones yet. He was not quite 145. Pounds. Though at times it definitely felt like years.

On the next Greenwich clinic visit he was tested with Tensilon, found to be underdosed, and the Mestinon was jacked up a wee bit. Next day, when it was evident that wasn't doing much good, they decided to use adjunctives.

The myasthenic reacted badly to the potassium experiment. Ephedrine failed to increase fading muscle strength. They went back to boosting the Mestinon. Slowly. But up.

The trach-tube had to be changed every couple of days. Somewhere, during one of these replacements, the bugs got in under the door and his trachea became infected. That tied him to the house for three days until they were able to clear it up. Then, just before November bowed off the calendar, there came a crisis. Breathing again. Labored. Swallowing went haywire shortly thereafter in one fell swoop and of course he aspirated. Spasms. Rush to the hospital. Plug in the respirator. Push down the goddamned tube. Put him back in his old care room up in ICU. Stand by for the fourth ACTH course, which lasted from November 30 to two days before Christmas.

Number four turned out to be as rugged as its forebears. But it is the happy nature of the human animal to wash out much of life's disagreeables. As he regained strength and the intercostals went back to work, the torments of that debilitating therapy seemed eminently worth the while.

The sick man did better on this course than on any of the others. He'd been taking 13 cc. of Mestinon when he went into the course. Every four hours, for 78 a day. Now he had been reduced to 7 cc.; then 3; then none. For nearly five days, no drugs at all! An amazing development. He soared as he thought that some mysterious combination had come up on the wheel and— God spare the thought—he had been cured. Not for long, that gaudy dream. The muscles began to poop out again and they saw it as prudent to put a little—less than 2 cc. to begin with—into the old pot again.

Now came some surgery he hadn't counted on. Mother Nature didn't fancy that hole in his throat and was setting about closing it. As the stoma was shrunk by the body's own recuperative machinery, it became difficult and painful to take the tracheostomy-tubes in and out of his throat. So a piece of the trachea had to be cut away and the triangular edges of the wound split back upon themselves and sewn so that the hole would remain open. They used a local. It was not money for jam.

The symptoms were held in check for several weeks after he'd come home from the hospital, and while the swallowing muscles were operating at 100 percent of capacity, they were strong enough for him to put down, with appropriate murmurs of appreciation, the excellent duck dinner Doris had prepared for Christmas. Could she cook! Sheer joy was the succulent sauce for such fine people-food. And what in the world could be tastier than a St. Ivel's plum pudding and hard sauce?

New Year's Eve was a delightful celebration. He and his wife and daughter drove down the Connecticut Turnpike into Manhattan to The Players for dinner, auld langs, and champagne at the witching hour.

He was aware that he must be filling out a little. Looking better. Certainly he was feeling better. A gaggle of his fellow members, drinks in hand in the Great Hall of Edwin Booth's one-time home, mock-solemnly agreed that he ought to get a new writer. He ought to have a new role to play. The part he'd been playing, they said, the desperately ill, sympathy-fetching, beloved old terminal case—well, it had been played out, they said. He'd milked it dry. It was over, now. Kapoot. Fee-nee.

"No question about it, pal," one of them said. "A good writer can fix you up with another part in no time. But you gotta do something besides that old invalid bit. Sheesh!"

"Yep, that sick role has been played out," said another.

"Played to the hilt," Roland Winters remarked.

"And beyond," his wife put in quietly.

They roared. And couldn't have loved her more.

Happy New Year!

CHAPTER 10

◆§ Throw a lucky man into the sea and he will come up with a fish in his mouth.—Arabian proverb

THE happy state that gala evening ushered in did not persist. Relief from the strictures of paralyzed muscles was short-lived. In less than three weeks he was in trouble again. Throat, mainly. On two occasions he aspirated. The first one was disagreeable but not explosive. The other one sent him into a body-jarring paroxysm that lasted nearly twenty minutes and thoroughly wrung him out.

By the middle of February he was in serious trouble. ACTH had been tried for the fourth time and for the fourth time it had failed more than temporary relief. If this was to be the pattern, the sick man didn't see any more ACTHs in his future. Surely there was something else. But even as he mouthed the hope, minor despair engulfed him. What choice was there? The experts seemed to agree that ACTH was the best therapy for myasthenia.

It was here that the gods smiled.

Dr. Walter Camp, the Greenwich neurologist who had diagnosed his disease, agreed that ACTH didn't seem to hold much promise for his patient.

"I've been thinking a lot about it," he told the worried man. "There's a research program we might get you into, if you'd like to try it. They've gotten some good results so far."

"I'll try anything. Tell me about it."

As part of a continuing neuromuscular research program, myasthenia gravis was currently under study at the National Institute of Neurological Diseases and Stroke, one of the components of the huge National Institutes of Health complex in Bethesda.

A coincidence of great improbability had taken place. Four diverse elements—doctor, disease, patient, project—had had to come together neatly at the same time. The doctor had to know about the NINDS program. (Since he had served as deputy to Dr. King Engel, chief of the Medical Neurology Branch of NINDS, Dr. Camp was fully familiar with myasthenia.) Next, the disease had to be under study at that particular time. (It was.) The patient's case had to be a virulent one, in a man of an age the scientists wanted to work on. (The Connecticut myasthenic filled the bill admirably.) So, when his case was described by Dr. Camp and he was suggested as a candidate, they said they'd clear a bed for him as soon as they could.

He went on home to wait. He was going to be guinea pig number three in a new and specialized neuromuscular project in which the first two patients had done surprisingly well. Heartened, he slept well that night and rose to a bright morning. But toward noon he hit a downdraft. Symptoms rapidly increased in severity. When the chest muscles began to stumble, his wife phoned the doctor and delivered her husband to Greenwich Hospital. They put him to bed.

During the early months of that year, the sick man had kept daily notes of his condition and how he had reacted to his medication. It couldn't be said with any accuracy that these memoranda were as exciting as an Eric Ambler spy story, but they did represent a fair pattern of what went on in the life of a myasthenic whose muscles frequently went so weak it would have been foolhardy for him to challenge an effeminate katydid.

Apart from giving him something constructive to do, the diary notes on his reactions to the various drug dosages were useful to the doctors. And there was always the hope that one day, when his case had bottomed out and been buttoned up, the notes might provide some answers for future researchers.

Characteristic of the roller-coaster nature of his malady, his dose of Mestinon was at the surprisingly low point of 1 cc. a day. It held him on balance for a few days and then had to be increased to bolster sagging muscles. When they boosted it to three times a day, it turned out to be a mistake. Perversely, the drug degenerated the muscles instead of strengthening them, as it always had done before. The doctors were as baffled by the phenomenon as he was.

Two days later he had materially improved. The very next day he turned south again. It was all very confusing. And that's the way it went—up hill and down dale—throughout the entire month. They upped the dosage, little by little, with careful watch against the dangerous overdose. Even so, by mid-February he was up to 12 cc. five times a day. That's 60 cubic centimeters of Mestinon, which comes to 720 milligrams of anticholinesterase a day, a great deal more than he was taking at the beginning of the year. It was beginning to look as if he might be losing the war.

The next day, shortly after he had finished lunch, which was fairly tasty as hospital meals go, both his breathing and his swallowing muscles began to fade rapidly. It didn't take them long to jab a tube through his nose so they could get food and medicine into his stomach. Then they wheeled in a Bird respirator and its oxygen cylinder and plugged him into it. His roommate, recovering from third-degree burns, found the activity and the machinery fascinating. The myasthenic was considerably less beguiled.

The smells, the sounds, the uncomfortable and confining tubes sharply tried his patience almost before he'd warmed the bed. He damned the circumstances that had delivered him once more to a hospital room. Bad luck. More than he felt he should be made to suffer. It was just this side of weepy. Happily the saving grace came to the rescue. Only a fool kicks the tire when it goes flat. There comes a time when a man has to sit it out with his hands quietly in his lap.

The next nine days crawled by. Most of the time with his hands in his lap. He was readjusting. Again. And then, on the Friday, along about the time the western light was beginning to change and the trees on the sharp-rising bluff across the way were going dusty purple, Dr. Camp walked briskly into the room. He was smiling. Broadly.

On Sunday, the seventh of March, 1971, the myasthenic set out with his wife, a nurse, a breathing-machine, and a hope on a long, uncomfortable, immensely welcome journey.

CHAPTER 11

◄§ *The art of medicine consists of three things: the disease,
the patient, the physician. The patient must combat the disease
along with the physician.*—Hippocrates

THE ambulance was fifty-odd miles from Bethesda when it came time for feeding and medication. The nurse set about the task with the easy grace of the pro. She poured the light-brown formula into the gavage bag, hung it from a ceiling hook, and lifted the nose-tube off the patient's left ear. The foot-long piece of soda-straw-sized plastic tube sticking out of his nose was a nuisance when it wasn't in use. Best way to keep it out of the way was to drape it over an ear.

Nurse pulled the plug out of the end of the tube, inserted the tip of the plungerless syringe, flushed the tube with a little water, and, without spilling a drop, sent the cherry-colored Mestinon down into his stomach.

Inasmuch as he was on the respirator, the cuff of the trach-tube was already inflated, pressing the little rubber doughnut against the inner walls of the trachea and blocking the passage of air above the stoma, the hole in his throat through which the trach-tube protruded. The paper-thin cuff could be deflated at will, as was done when he was able to breathe on his own, but usually it was kept inflated to let nothing but air get into the windpipe and bronchial tubes.

A splash of water cleared the syringe of the thin, red film so that every bit of the drug would get into his system. The gavage-bag tube was plugged in, the clamp eased off, and the liquid meal began to flow. The formula had been contrived to supply two thousand calories a day and consisted of milk, eggs, strained meat, pureed fruits, fruit juices, and vitamins. Despite its unappetizing appearance, the lightly viscous liquid didn't have a disagreeable taste, as he thought it might, when he sampled it later on. But it wasn't likely to be mistaken for vintage port.

After each meal it was important to flush the tube thoroughly so that the formula wouldn't harden and clog it. That had happened to him once, at Mt. Sinai Hospital. The floor doctor had to be summoned. Out came the stopped-up tube and a fresh one shoved through already irritated nose and throat. Not the end of the world but not much fun, either.

This wasn't the only peril in tube-feeding. There was one booby trap that was a dilly. Sometimes the nurse wasn't as careful as she might have been and so failed to hold the tip of the large syringe securely into the end of the nasogastric tube during feeding. Without the right amout of restraint when the syringe is filled with formula, the tip of the tube can easily slip out, cascading the gooey mess all over patient and bed in a thick, brown flood.

How the cleanup was handled depended on the nurse and on how much activity there was on the ward at the time. There might be no more than perfunctory mop-up, with the bed left messy-damp until next linen-change. Or there could be a thorough body-wash, a new johnny-coat or fresh PJs and clean bed linen. But even then, weak and uncomfortable, the patient didn't welcome being rolled back and forth while the bed-change was being carried on. It wasn't painful but it was definitely uncomfortable.

Still, he wryly told himself, it could be worse and it did break up the monotony.

Oh yes, there's another tube-feeding chore. Checking for stomach residuals. At the better-regulated institutions, and the 5-East Ward at the Clinical Center certainly qualified, it was *de rigueur* to insert a collapsed syringe into the NG-tube and draw the plunger out slowly, bringing with it whatever liquids were in the stomach, for checking. Too much of the goop and the tube-feeding had to be delayed until digestion broke it down and the pyloric stomach valve waved it on its way to the small intestine.

The residuals, he had observed, were almost always a gay, yellowish color. How the ends of the NG-tubes, when they'd been snaked out of him, got so black he never could figure out.

CHAPTER 12

✍ *Try all things. Hold to that which is good.* —*1 Thessalonians*

LATE on the afternoon of that March 7, the ambulance pulled out of the stream of traffic onto a quiet road winding itself through rolling lawns just coming awake after the winter cold. Dogwoods, pine, and magnolia made the low brick buildings that clustered around the imposing, multistoried Clinical Center seem less severe.

The ambulance circled the building and backed into the curb. Inside, the nurse spread an extra blanket over her patient, checked his need for suctioning, and, as the car doors opened, disconnected the respirator hose and inserted the nozzle of an ambu into his trach-tube. The easy, rhythmic squeezing forced air in and out of his lungs, just as the mechanical breathing-machine had been doing throughout the three-hundred-mile journey.

When the orderlies pulled the stretcher out and set it on its wheels on the pavement, the sick man had the odd sensation that he was not a stranger to this place, though he knew he had never been there before. He was sharply struck, for all of the misery of the moment, with the certainty that he'd gone through the same routine at another time. It was not *déjà vu* and he knew he had never seen Bethesda before. Yet this antic of his mind disturbed him out of all proportion to the importance of the event. Sometimes the seriously ill see strange ghosts.

Quickly they wheeled him out of the chill, raw day into a warm hall that gave onto the elevators. On the fifth floor they turned him into the care room, directly opposite the nurses' station, where he'd be always under their eye. When they'd settled him in, his wife went off to talk with the floor doctor who would be looking after her husband. After they'd plugged him into the respirator, all but the duty nurse turned to other tasks. A final check to see that all was in order and she let him rest. He had arrived at his laboratory. Guinea pig number three.

There is no satisfactory laboratory animal for myasthenia gravis, he'd been told. The myasthenic himself must serve. And as the sick man saw himself in that role, a ten-year-old piece of memory was thrown onto the screen by his mnemonic projector.

In that old yesterday he had been researching a magazine article, which called for a visit to a laboratory in New Jersey that was using small animals to test the products of a cosmetics company. The visit had been abortive from the start. Not only wasn't he getting the information he wanted but he'd taken an instant, ten-gallon dislike to his guide, a scruffy, rat-faced man in a dirty smock. On top of that, he was upset at seeing the cooped animals in their too-small, stacked cages. The judgment button was pressed heavily. Plain to see that rat-face was a sadist who, when he was not neglecting his charges, mistreated them. Moreover, it was equally obvious that he fiddled the time clock, was slovenly on his job, and had disgusting eating habits. No point in taking one's dislikes too lightly.

By now the fetid room was heavily oppressive. He hurried his inspection, wanting nothing so much as to leave the place. As he made to do so, he was prodded to make some kind of protest against this use of living animals. He was as startled as his guide when, turning at the door, he called out in a strident voice to the cages, "Hang in there, fellows."

At once he was flushed with remorse for that impertinent exhortation. There was no hope for those little beasts. The phrase was veined with cruelty. Thinly, perhaps, but it was there, out of his thoughtlessness. As he left the room, his stomach had the good grace to churn disagreeably.

Here in his Bethesda hospital room he felt as caged as those laboratory animals of a decade ago. He, like them, would be given strange drugs and his reactions would be checked and charted. And, as with them, there were no open options. But his predicament was far from hopeless. It was definitely a time to heed his own admonition and hang in there.

There were two dozen patients on the 5-East Ward when all the beds were filled. The rooms accommodated two beds comfortably, although his had only one. It was a spacious room in spite of all the gear that was in it. The high window opened to the south. The slotted blinds had to be closed at night to keep the sun from playing alarm clock. On the right, coming into the room, were the toilet and bath. The toilet seat had been built up four or five inches, like platform shoes, so that there wouldn't be too much strain on weak and flaccid muscles getting on and off. On the rack above the fire-engine red emergency button, which would bring help on the double, were stacked graduated metal vessels for measuring urine output, stool-sample containers, placards to remind the patient to do or not to do this or that, and sundry other items rarely found any place other than hospital bathrooms.

In the room itself, to the right, sharing a wall with the bath, were two metal clothes lockers and a recessed washbasin with mirror and towel racks. To the left, the two squat, three-drawered oaken Formica chests had been pushed together to form a single unit. Their tops were burdened with bottles and boxes and small instruments. The drawers were filled with hospital linen, the patient's personal impedimenta, and a mélange of oddments nobody ever got around to using. In one of the bottom drawers was a thick, wooled sheepskin, which warmed the myasthenic in those early days when it seemed he was perpetually cold.

There were two respirators in the room. The Bennett, quietly pulling oxygen out of the wall and sending it into his lungs, was backstopped by a Bird respirator, a smaller machine that didn't run for him as smoothly as the Bennett. No matter. The Bird was comforting insurance. Another demonstration of the thoroughness of the staff planning. And there was further insurance in the black rubber ambu that perched on top of the oxygen outlet above his bed. Power failure couldn't cut off the vital supply of air to the ailing.

The several metal tables in the room, some containing lift tops that covered small mirrors and inset trays for personal toiletries, were piled high with catheters and dressings, bottles of distilled water for the respirator's humidifier, rubber gloves, swabs and gauze patches, adhesive tapes, and plastic cups filled with lemon swabs. It is indeed the little things that count. Paralyzed face muscles prevented him from washing his teeth or sloshing water around in his mouth to freshen it. Those wonderful lemon swabs solved the problem.

Beyond the foot of the bed, which could be raised and lowered mechanically (an Olympian boon to the nurse when she had to change the linen) was the television set. The small hand-console was pinned at his right side, where he could reach the buttons that turned the ad-padded mind-boggler on and off, changed channels and volume. On his left, hand-high, was pinned the console whose buttons moved the bed into a number of comfort-making configurations. Feet up, feet down. Knees up, knees down. The right amount of up-feet and up-knees, with whatever up-back was required, would produce a declivity for the arse parts that prevented slipping lower and lower in the bed to the point where he had to yell for help and two nurses had to come in, take positions on either side of him, lock under his arms and, by the numbers, haul him back up with a jolly heave-ho. They invariably puffed and positioned the pillows. They didn't half make him comfortable. He'd never been made more so in his life.

It was getting late now. It had been a busy day. He was tired. The night nurse, who moved in a ponderous way and looked like the movies' Hattie McDaniel in the beam, rocked to the demands of her bunions as she walked. With a gentleness the big fingers might not be suspected of, she pressed his arm to reassure him as she came to the bed, rubber-gloved herself and sucked the secretions out of his chest. She smiled down at him, three gold-cased front teeth catching the light.

"You'll do jes' fine," she said, softly. "Get a good night. Hear?"

She turned down the lights and took her seat at the little table against the far wall to do her paper work and watch over him until midnight, when her relief came on.

The soft sobbing of the breathing-machine was all that stirred the silence. Singularly secure, the myasthenic closed his eyes and was gone. He did have a good night.

The first few days were occupied with tests, proddings, questions, observations. There were blood samplings and X-rays, repeated blowing into silver instruments that looked like king-size police whistles, to check the vital lung capacity. There was a large aluminum device to squeeze so that hand-grip or lack of it could be measured. He was hammer-tapped at various body junctures to make leg kicks or feet flexings. And there was one session where there were needle jabs to find out if he could feel the pricking. He could. This was as close to acupuncture as they ever got, except for the EMG, the electromyogram, which was much more dramatic, with fluttery lines flashing on oscillographic screens to the accompaniment of buzzings and wheezings and once in a while some startling thumps.

It was heartening to see that the patients in this ward weren't looked upon as if they were studying to be cretins. The doctors talked to them as less-informed peers, patiently explaining, patiently satisfying anxious curiosity. The chief of the Medical Neurology Branch, his deputy, and the floor doctor converged on the myasthenic almost every day to tell him as clearly as they could how they regarded his particular affliction, how they proposed to treat it, and why it was necessary, straight away, to take him off all drugs before beginning their own therapeutic program.

This was the fifth cold-turkey withdrawal from the cholinergic drug he had been taking ever since his disease had been diagnosed. It wasn't any easier this time. The ten days between his admission to NIH and the first dose of prednisone was a little on the hairy side. He got a lot weaker, he thought, than on earlier withdrawals. And while he was strung tight out physically, mentally he was sharp as the razor's edge. His mind went galloping all over the place and he was more than frustrated that he couldn't ask all of the questions that crowded into his head. He thought a good deal about the new drug. Just what was prednisone? What would it do to him? How soon would it take effect? What would the side effects be like?

In Greenwich, when he and Dr. Camp had first talked about the NIH program, there had been references to the drug that were a little like one of those "I've got good news and bad news" jokes. The good news was that prednisone had already cured or almost cured two people. The bad news was that the side effects included bleeding ulcers, bone calcium loss, cataracts, high blood pressure, fluid retention in body tissues, heart failure, insomnia, nervousness, and rare cases of cork-popping psychosis.

So what? It isn't too safe to cross a busy street these days, he reassured himself. The good news so far outwarmed the bad that he saw himself already in the winner's circle. Later, when the prednisone had worked its miracle on him and none of the dire side effects had appeared, he was reaffirmed in his belief that we fret far more than we need to.

On the morning of St. Patrick's Day in 1971 he was given his first dose of prednisone. Nothing happened. Somehow he was disappointed. Bending his mind to it, it was easy to see that the drug was not likely to produce frothing at the mouth or any of the divine, dramatic reactions such as rising up from the dead or picking up the bed and walking. Still, he insisted, there should have been some signal, shouldn't there? Maybe prednisone wasn't all that potent, after all. Impatience again. He curbed it.

Prednisone was not a newly discovered wonder drug. Its value lay in how it was used, in what doses, in what time frame, in combination with what other chemicals. And how the patient tolerated it.

The myasthenic's London doctor, experienced in myoneurology for many years, had used this particular drug early in his practice in treating myasthenia gravis and had rejected it. It had failed to produce the hoped-for results. Apparently Dr. Greene had not used the chemical in large enough quantities over long enough periods of time. Or perhaps his patients had been unsympathetic to this potent drug, which smiles so benignly when the right dose, the right time, and the right patient come together. When such a meeting occurs, happy day!

Prednisone, like a number of artificial steroids, was derived from cortisone in the 1950s and used as an inflammation-suppressant in such ailments as rheumatoid arthritis. The liver converts this artificial steroid into prednisolone, and that directly spurs the adrenal glands to make the hormones the body requires. Prednisone is convenient to use and it has a treatment record of dosages, established by good old trial and error.

Generally it is accepted that one hundred milligrams at forty-eight-hour intervals is about the right amount of drug to supply enough steroids to suppress disease symptoms without smothering the adrenals. This can be a serious problem. When the drug is administered several times daily, the adrenal glands don't have enough time to recover from overstimulation. So, after a period of repeated exhaustions, they cease to function altogether.

That 100-milligram figure isn't sacrosanct. The practitioner has to temper the dosage to the case in hand, in his own best judgment. At one point in his therapy, the Connecticut myasthenic was being given 175 milligrams alternating with 50. That quantity must have made the adrenal glands scream.

Perhaps the clankiest ghost that stalks the use of prednisone as treatment for myasthenia is that it eats up such an enormous amount of time. And time, in health care, translates into large sums of money.

Despite the relatively rapid recovery of the lead-off guinea pig in the prednisone project at NIH, the seven weeks of his treatment would have run up a crunching bill at a private hospital. It took number two in the old program three months to bring the muscles back to near-normal usability. The Greenwich man, number three, would spend twice that time and a little more before his miracle was brought to pass.

Not many these days are well-heeled enough to spend half a year in a hospital room. Not many can come up handily with that kind of scratch.

Those fortunate enough to be invited to bring their maladies to Bethesda for study, and possible cure, found the question academic. At the National Institutes there are no patient charges.

The National Institutes of Health is an organization devoted to medical research. It is housed in a cluster of fifty buildings, settled pleasingly to the eye on three hundred country acres a few miles north of the nation's capital city. It is the principal research arm of the Department of Health, Education and Welfare, which also supports research in medical and dental schools, and colleges and universities, abroad as well as in the United States.

NIH was born in a small laboratory at the Marine Hospital on Staten Island when Rutherford Birchard Hayes was President of the United States. It has grown considerably and today is manned by thirteen thousand men and women who possess some of the finest medical brains in the world. Doctors and scientists from every country seek entrance to this institution. Some of the young American doctors who are invited to the Clinical Center for special research training are given one year of floor service with the patients, and one year in the well-equipped laboratories.

The largest building is the Clinical Center, a fourteen-story research hospital with hundreds of labs crowded with the most modern, sophisticated machinery and equipment it is possible to come by and five hundred beds for the patients who are selected to participate in specific research projects.

Patient-welfare and research requirements go arm in arm at

the Clinical Center. Procedures that involve risk to the patient, and many of them do, are never undertaken until they are thoroughly explained and approved by the patient, no matter how important to the research project.

Alpha-and-omega records are compiled and maintained. This running recording requires that certain patients return periodically for tests and observations, just as the Connecticut myasthenic would be doing one day.

Applications for patient admission to NIH are made daily. Those pressed down by stubborn or exotic afflictions pray for a chance to submit themselves to the skills of the doctors and scientists of the institution. Many call but few are chosen. None buys a ticket. NIH is a research facility, aiming not to cure but to learn how to cure. Only when it seems likely to advance the knowledge of an obstinate disease is the door opened.

The Clinical Center roster is a congress of drastic and arcane maladies. Spastics, manics, terminals with unknown afflictions, unfortunates with brain tumors and spinal abnormalities, psychotics, epileptics, muscular distrophics, ataxics, contorted arthritics, victims of shaking palsy and quarter-ton obesity, and pitiable children rendered nearly hairless by radiation treatments.

Sweet Jesus, what a litany.

Minds and bodies more savagely beaten than are seen elsewhere in such deplorable concentration.

Nursing demands here are different in degree from those of the private hospitals. The ward work, exaggerated by the nature of the maladies under study and by their numbers, tends to depressive disposure much sharper than is to be found elsewhere. It is not a nursing cakewalk when newly arrived epileptics are deprived of their anticonvulsive medications, so that uninhibited tests can be made to determine the seat of their trouble. These tests, usually made preamble to surgery, are a guard against injury to vital nerve centers under the knife. But the body pays no attention to such precautions when it is seized. To see the victims, especially the young children, in the devil's arms, thrown about in demonic dance, is a horrendous experience.

After he had become ambulatory and before his release from the Clinical Center, the myasthenic from Connecticut became fairly well acquainted with sometimes unusual pressures on the staff. He was a prejudiced witness, but it seemed to him that there was more sympathetic concern, generally, in the NIH wards than he'd experienced in the private hospitals. He couldn't help but wonder if money might not be at the root of it. In all the months he spent at Bethesda, and he had done a bit of prying, he had never been privy to even a casual wage complaint. And certainly none of the patients, unlike those he had observed in the hospitals in New York, were worried by mountainous medical costs.

·

CHAPTER 13

The three natural anesthetics are fainting, sleep, death.—Oliver Wendell Holmes

MYASTHENIA gravis is a very expensive disease.

The costs of treating this malady range as widely as its fluctuating symptoms. The sick man's first hospital tour, in Manhattan, stretched to nearly thirty days. There was surgery —thymectomy and tracheostomy—for which the fee was $1,000. Use of the operating room, anesthetic services, and kindred costs broke the back of another thousand.

The Intensive Care Unit, way station after the Recovery Room ($125), where he had gone through his first cold-turkey drug withdrawal, was billed at $225 a day. Next stop was the General Care Ward, where beds, in four-bedded rooms, were charged at $90 each. (Two years later these same "semiprivate" beds would be up to $115 and $120, and private beds would be $165.)

These charges are basic. Everything else is extra, including medications, oxygen, laboratory services, doctors' fees, and the morning newspaper. In New York, the doctor charged $40 a hospital visit (now up as high as $60). In Greenwich, it was $25. It has since gone up in the suburbs, too.

The myasthenic had been in the hospital in New York from April 26 to May 22. The bill came to nearly $8,000. His second ACTH course, in the same hospital, ran from June 20 to July 10, and came in at a little more than half that. There were no charges for surgery this time.

His third and fourth ACTH courses, administered in the Greenwich Hospital, cost about $3,500 each, which was lower than the big-city rates but still enough to wound the bank account.

The economic skeleton of such brushes with ill-health is roughly $250 a day, $7,500 a month, $90,000 a year. Additional costs are numerous. Private nursing care, required around the clock when the myasthenic is on artificial respiration, comes to $125 a day. Prednisone tablets, with 5 milligrams of the drug, are available in group and other special pharmacies for $3 to $4 a hundred. But when the prescribed dose is around 150 milligrams, those few dollars' worth don't go very far. Regular drug stores, even the cut-rates, charge nearly three times that price. All in all, the various adjunctives, the antacid and the vitamin pills so many doctors are prescribing, can run from $90 to $125 or $150 a month.

Prednisone lets potassium (K) leak out of the body in the urine. It must be replaced. Too little K and muscles begin to fail, especially the intercostals, which take care of breathing. Too much K can act as a brake on the heart, although excess potassium is eliminated with other body wastes. The kidneys are supposed to take care of that. In any case, when the chemical has to be supplied, the friendly druggist (on prescription) will provide a small bottle, enough for a week or so, at $6 to $9. Potassium comes in effervescent tablets at a couple of dollars a dozen. Usual dosage is two a day. Five grams. These bubbly tablets are potassium *citrate*. One has to be sure to take enough potassium *chloride*, which is usually prepared in syrup form. The British make potassium tablets called "Slow-K," but American doctors say they can burn holes in the bowels, because they are enteric-coated, pass unaltered through the stomach into the gut, and then disintegrate. Whether or not there is a tinge of chauvinism in this view, our doctors frown on "Slow-K."

Silver tracheostomy tubes seem to be more comfortable to most myasthenics than the plastic jobs, but the cuffs have a short life and it isn't easy to get a satisfactory recuffing done. The silver tubes cost around $20; plated tubes are some $5 less; plastic tubes, which can be used for several days before being discarded, cost $6 to $8, depending on the medical-supply house one deals with.

But all such costs as these are dwarfed drastically by the reckoning for the Connecticut myasthenic's care at the Clinical Center had it been charged at going rates. With the help of a fellow patient and two veteran nurses, he toted up twenty-four-hour nursing care, medications, X-ray and laboratory services, special equipment use, private room, attention of as many as seven scientist/specialists, various services—the works: $500 a day! And that was a modest calculation. Accepting that figure, the sick man's tour from March 7 to August 10 would run up a tab of $15,000 a month. Total for that confinement: $91,000.

Apply these numbing numbers to the myasthenics who must hobble along for years without remission and they begin to lose a sense of reality. The sick man knew of five myasthenics in the New York area each of whom had carried his burden for more than fifteen years.

Myasthenia is not alone among man's bodily woes but it is, among other things, hell on the wallet.

Calculations of the cost of medical care in the private sector helped sharpen the sick man's unenthusiastic attitude toward medicine in general into bias. He knew better than to allow himself to wallow in bloc prejudices. Such aberrations, in any form, rasped against convictions he'd held since he was a small boy; certainly since his discovery of general semantics, his first understanding that the map is not the territory, and that selective intolerance is as valid as it is necessary to existence in modern society. He had found the most sensible idea the simplest one: accept man one, woman one. Reject man two, woman two. Hug child one; smack child two. Individual selectivity. No group lump.

He was fanned by his own medical experiences and this made him tend to see doctors as a group through jaundiced eyes. The notable exceptions emphasized the opinion. He was tempered, too, by the long-held dislike of *having* to go to the doctor and *having* to take pills and elixirs. There were times when one couldn't avoid the medical man, as when, in his early days, he acquired a forest of carbuncles on the back of his neck. There was nothing for it but the knife. Later on, with a hernia, he didn't fancy doing the hem-stitching himself, so there was a short hospital stay for that repair.

But now, despite dislike of pills and their prescribers, he took concoctions with as little fuss as possible. He didn't want to come up helpless on his back. But he never did get over wishing he didn't have to take the medicines.

Almost from the day he had applied to the hospital in New York for admission, he was put off by what seemed to him to be a callous air of unconcern for the patient as an individual. Not that one might expect the greetings oilionaires are given at the grand hotels. But the hospital staff attitude seemed to be a kind of pecking-order broth of arrogance and self-importance. Some of the young men, now learning their craft or just serving their time, would set up shop in fashionable neighborhoods and call on other than medical skills in the presence of monied matrons. The carriage trade is not to be found in the general wards. And other of these incipient practitioners would carry throughout their careers an abhorrence of the terminally ill that would diminish them as doctors. They would see the doomed as the patients to be avoided whenever it could be done safely, or as their own personal failures. Not by numbers but by other yardsticks they may well have been outweighed by those of their fellows who saw more than the dying body and were compassionately impelled to give full dignity and ease to death.

Hospitals are factories for treating, training, and dying. It is deplorable when less than competence and honesty are provided. The sick man rarely missed a chance to preach this gospel.

Deplorable, he'd say, in argumentative heat even when nary a contra word had been spoken. Deplorable. Makes a fellow cynical. Makes him agree that them as has, gits. And that there is truth in the ancient waggish crack that the only thing money can't buy is poverty.

For all the green that flows into Medicine Pond, more attention than they sometimes get is due those who come to the hospital door. Odious and offensive patients are not easy pills for anyone to swallow, but none of the halt and ailing need be brushed off. So very often they are. He had incidents supporting this contention.

Minor: On three occasions the patient was asked a professional question during a bed-call, only to have the interlocutor, in the middle of the response, turn full attention to something or someone else.

Major: The myasthenic was allowed to go a full three days without a bowel movement, despite repeated complaints. Not one of the Nightingales seemed interested enough to see that it was taken care of. Not until he was severely impacted did a rubber glove go on. Then, after two ineffectual but messy enemas (a practice expressly forbidden for myasthenics because of the weakening effects of the sluicings), it was hell's delight having the waste pried out of him.

If there was ever a time he wanted to ask the doctor, in a loud and carrying voice, how much malpractice time he had put in, that was it. But the moment flew off on the wings of cowardice and the pearl was never dropped. When he did complain, not at all in the clever, ingenious way he'd hoped it would be, he was told with condescending impatience to knock off the bitching, which is what was said even though other words were used. One nurse lost her popularity standing by reminding the sick man how much better off he was than some of the other patients.

The lust for blood went up another couple of notches at that. On the one hand, it is drab to make such irrelevant comparisons. Is a man's broken leg improved by the fact of two fractures of the femur in the neighboring bed? On the other, it's a put-down.

The myasthenic's illiberal views may not have been the most just judgments. The sample was small, for one; and for two, the practitioners at Greenwich and Bethesda tipped the scales with no mean weight. He was not alone in his jaundiced attitude toward the profession. Shocking revelations were related by friends. Daily the public prints reported medical incompetence, venality, and questionable practices. To be sure, the good news seldom rings the chimes as loudly as the bad, but the myasthenic demanded a better average when it came to care and cure. Which made it understandable that, determined to flog his disapprovals unmercifully, he recalled with stern disapproval the three times he had seen the cream-colored Cadillac with the MD plates, widely double-parked in front of the Grand Union market in his neighborhood. He gave this civic sin unusual weight. After he'd eyed the opulent shopping cart for the third time, he muttered darkly to himself, "But no damned house calls."

Since this isn't a strictly two-toned world, the myasthenic conceded a minim of value in the no-house-call edict, though he did entertain a special disapproval of it. The medical advocates' blanket insistence that it was no longer a practical practice was a Swiss-cheese argument.

"When somebody complains of chest pains, what do you do? We can't carry EKG machines around in our little black bags."

"Those wee-hour calls can get sticky. We're sitting ducks for the addicts and the muggers."

Such contentions covered too much ground. Not all calls for the doctor's visit are for chest pains and there are effective defenses against being rapped on the occiput on a dark street. The practitioner's receiving patients, however ill, at his office, does give him more time to see more people. Gives him more time for golf, too.

It is a puzzlement at best. When the demand end outweighs the supply end, inequities abound. Doctors these days are in short supply. It may have been only a wild-eyed Abyssinian hunch, but the myasthenic was pretty sure this short supply was more than a happenstance.

This less than rosy view had not been brightened by the Associated Press report that the American Medical Association had accepted $10 million from the tobacco industry for "research." The published findings were predictable: "Any evidence that smoking is bad for the health is inconclusive." This kind of arrant nonsense must have been one of the spurs that goaded some of the fifteen thousand who resigned from the AMA out of those hallowed halls.

Lab tests and X-rays are eyebrow-raisers, too. Many are utter waste, ordered more often because they have always been ordered than for diagnostic need. And since divergent results are read from the same tests and films, there may be a ferret in this hen house. One thing persists: no question where the charges go.

The consultant call cuts two ways. Useful, when specialist opinion is actually required. Abused, when there are referral understandings and when doctors are unwilling to make unbackstopped diagnoses.

This is not the Rock Candy Mountains side of medicine. The ailant and his family have to make the best of it. It's the only wheel in town. As in other pursuits in this best of all possible worlds, incompetence and carelessness strut onto the stage, and the love that is said to be the root of all evil is the most likely candidate for the lion's share of blame for this perversion. Those in medicine who do their work in conscientious honesty sharply point up their arrant siblings and make it evident that no civilized society will allow the money ethic to dominate matters of life and death.

Hospital staffs are villains of the piece, too.

People sicker than hell have stumbled into admission offices and, unable to convince the help that they could cover the tab, were not led with tender loving care to a bed for treatment. Cost cards at many hospitals carry a caveat: If you are not covered by hospital insurance, a deposit of $1,500 will be required at time of admission.

Of course, before financial matters can come up on the agenda, the applicant has to be noticed. On two occasions, the sick man himself had been required to wait much longer than was necessary to fill up the forms. It isn't all that difficult to tell when the normal pressures of work slow down personal attention or whether delay is the result of customer unconcern. Attitude is a fairly reliable signpost.

In his first application for admission, so weak he tottered, the clerk gave more attention to an animated social conversation with her seatmate than to the job at hand. On the second occasion, the young lady got up and went away in the middle of the form-filling exercise, with nary a word, and never did come back. Call of nature, maybe, or an early lunch.

Such incidents were less than mild irritants when seen against the *New York Times* report of the businessman, Reginald Foster, who had been rushed to hospital in desperate condition. He had been refused admission until he'd been able to provide financial guarantee. The delay was significant. He died six days later. His widow was presented with a $12,000 bill.

Toward the end of 1970's November, the myasthenic tried to make some sense out of the two bills that the hospital on Fifth Avenue had given him. Itemized copies were not easy to come by. His repeated requests to the hospital were ignored. Even when his doctor asked that copies be sent him, it took a few pounds of prodding to get the bouillabaisse of errors.

Review of the billings raised questions. None of his letters, asking for explanations, produced response. Telephone calls were fuzzed with double-talk.

Why, he had asked, did special nursing charges vary from $116 to $160 a day? The base period was twenty-four hours; the shared-patient charge could not account for the $44 spread.

Why, when he was in the ICU ward for two days, during a strike threat, was he also charged for special-duty nurses on the General Care Ward?

Why was he charged $105.75 for certain medications that brought single dose cost to $7, while a $24 charge for the same medicine, administered a smaller number of times, brought the unit dose charge to $2?

Why were different charges and duplicate charges made for the same quantities of the same medication, on five different occasions?

Why were charges for Mestinon on two given dates duplicated on other tallysheets for the same dates?

How come oxygen and artificial respirators were charged for six days during which the patient was breathing comfortably on his own?

How come X-ray charges during the first ACTH course were $300 higher than those for the second tour, although both courses were almost identical in treatment?

Some of the answers to these questions might have been quite reasonable. He never found out. Three years after his first letter of inquiry, despite repeated telephonic promises of competent response, nary an answer had been forthcoming. The myasthenic concluded that this was not bookkeeping at its best.

As he stirred the kettle of other people's sins, the distortions became abundantly clear. It was hardly his exclusive discovery that some medical types shouldn't be members of the club. Neither should some plumbers, priests, superior court judges, and bookmakers.

His affair with major medicine to date had hardly been a disaster. It hadn't all been beer and skittles but he'd been given what he'd been rapidly running out of—time. And the promise of a better than even chance to regain that other high desirable —muscle mobility.

He wasn't bored with the waiting for the miracle. Especially at the Clinical Center. When he wasn't being diagnostically thumped and prodded, there were vital signs and radiographic pictures to be taken. EKG and frequent EMG sessions were sandwiched with progress-photo sittings. Measurements of body intake and output were taken around the clock. There were pills and elixirs and syrups at frequent intervals. And every hour on the hour, or so it seemed, blood was being drawn for who knows how many different kinds of tests. Busy, busy needles.

But no serious complaints. Heaven forfend that the star should cavil. There was no doubt but that he was the star of the piece. Else why would the doctors bring in those groups of visiting medicos to show off his progress and learnedly discuss his case? There is sweet satisfaction in being the center of attention.

Then it came time for the biopsy.

A biopsy involves snipping a chunk of flesh out of the living body and shoving it under a microscope for examination. After this minisurgery had been performed on him, the ordeal didn't sound like torture in the telling but it was no cakewalk in the doing.

What they did was they wheeled him into the operating room one sunny morning in May. Operating rooms are very theatrical. Dramatic expanse of white enamel, stainless steel, green linen. Surgical odds and ends glittering in the glare of high-powered lights that hung over the table they lifted him onto. It chuckled him mildly to think that if they'd brought him in to blaring martial music, with nubile majorettes high-kneeing it feverishly, the sterile flamboyance of that room would not have been dampened whit one.

The biopsic drill was to slice a wisp of muscle out of the left leg at mid-thigh. It hurt a little when the knife went in but that wasn't nearly as uncomfortable as his having to lie flat out with head unsupported. Secretions built up rapidly in mouth and throat. He started to gag. The nurses, not to complain on them, were primarily interested in their surgical duties and at first paid his sputterings no mind. A few wheezes later one of them did diagnose his trouble and tucked a folded towel under his head. The juices ran down his throat. Sweet relief. So he got through the ordeal in one piece, glad it was over.

Perhaps the best part of the whole deal came to light later on, when the young doctor who had wrought this surgical masterpiece took sensual delight that the incision had healed so well that even a searching eye would have been hard put to locate the site.

With the biopsy out of the way, the freshet of tests tapered off. It was just as well. No need to sit in a corner with nothing to do but mope. He was almost breathless (figuratively speaking, of course) keeping on his toes. The Clinical Center provided a generous calendar of activities to beguile even the bored and brooding mind. During his tour, the myasthenic sampled most of the doings.

Every Friday, the patients' library cart, with excellent selections, called on patient rooms. Red Cross volunteers cheerfully offered to run errands and do in-town shopping. And every couple of weeks, a handsome, white-haired woman would bring around framed prints of fine art to brighten the walls.

There were movies twice a week—adult and family— bus tours into Washington for baseball games and visits to public buildings, and once in a while a special event, like Las Vegas Night, with poker, blackjack, chuck-a-luck, and roulette.

But during the time the myasthenic had been immobilized, it

hadn't been very gay. Accepting that he was ill and needed help, it was galling nonetheless when he tried to do a simple thing for himself and failed to bring it off. It was especially disagreeable when he felt his dignity had been compromised, as when he could see, with concentrated distaste, the scrawny, wasted, old-man body they lifted onto the bedpan. And his inability to hold his water, with the urinal on the way. It was one of the less dangerous but uncomfortably embarrassing side effects of his drugs.

The eliminatory functions bothered him most. Probably a Puritan inheritance. And he was offended by the grotesque postures his body fell into, in bed and out. He despised the days they came in to weigh him, when he was flaked out in bed. The orderlies would lift Old Scrawn out of bed like a slab of beef and plunk him down on the horizontal scale-bed, his head flopping about painfully until one of the nurses moved a pillow into place.

That weighing machine was as diabolical as Procrustes's bed. It was a vomitous example of industrial design at its nadir, to boot. There appears to be a fiction rampant in medical circles that this tortuous device would actually register poundage or kilograms of those patients who were too weak to stand on the upright scales. Ha ha, he sneered. The figure they come up with may just be in the ball park but that's about all it is.

It was after one of these weigh-ins, pinned again in bed by dormant muscles, and alone in his room, that the myasthenic saw his father in himself.

Almost forty years ago, in a Salt Lake City hospital, he had stood beside a bed like this, looking down at his father, who was stricken with a blasted heart. He could not remember what he had said or tried to say, if anything at all. They had looked at each other and were, as so often had been the case before, unable to reach each other when most they wanted to communicate.

The dying man's sallow, almost ashen face was startling in its contrast to the ruddy, sun-tanned countenance that had grinned merrily at him the last time they'd played golf together, when the tee shots were taking off on that true upward arc and the putts from the edge of the greens were going straight home every time.

For a long time they looked at each other. The younger man turned away to press his hand against his stepmother's flushed cheek, as she sat motionless a little distance from the bed.

When he returned his eyes to his father's face, he saw the

quivering around the lips and realized, almost with a sense of shock, what he'd known when he'd entered the room. His father could not speak. The misted eyes held a message the son could not read. He stared until, suddenly conscious of the futile survey, he looked guiltily away, avoiding the nurse's eyes, meeting his stepmother's. He smiled a wan, self-conscious smile that was instantly slaughtered. His father turned his head toward the wall. The young man said his good-byes almost silently. Nothing in the whole world had ever been so ineffectual as that farewell. The witches were stirring their acid brew in his stomach as he hurried out of the hospital.

A few blocks' walk, a passing cab, and he wound up three blocks from the railroad station, in a Temple Street saloon. He drank more whiskey than he was accustomed to, as he waited for the train that was to take him back to Los Angeles. The drink didn't seem to affect him very much.

He had made no arrangements for his father. He had been no comfort to his stepmother. He despised himself for this behavior. He had not wanted it to be that way. But there had been no inner struggle at the moment of decision. He simply could not have done other than he did. The visit to his father's deathbed had been an abject failure. He knew he would never see his father again. But he hadn't expected to see him again when, three years before, he had left Los Angeles to return to his old political-reporting job on the Salt Lake *Tribune*. The departure had not bothered the younger man then. Was it because of the presence of death that it bothered him now? Even as he asked he knew the answer didn't matter. Not a single thing could be changed.

Staring into the glass of tepid Scotch, he lighted a cigarette, ignoring the half-smoked Piedmont in the ash tray. Reflection on the past hour moved him almost to panic that he had so little control over himself. It was as if he had stood on a dizzying height and, crying out against the lemming action, had thrown himself into the abyss.

He shook his head in disbelief of the blank he drew. He could not remember a single incident prior to his standing at his father's bed. Whether he had come into Salt Lake by train or plane, where he had been living in Los Angeles, what he had been doing, how he had gotten word that his father was dying. Nothing. Not even the job he was waiting to go back to. Nothing. What blots out so much of our lives? And where does it go?

This black and dreadful mood eased up. He signaled for another drink, checked the clock, fired up another cigarette. He went back over the years to the young boy who had just arrived from Mobile to be brought up by his father and a new stepmother. Jessie did her best for him, but he had not been an easy boy to manage. Precocious enough to get passing grades with little effort, he went off into the fascinating worlds that grown people never knew about, his study books the only ones he didn't open.

A scene from the early days on East Third South blew a laugh loud enough to startle the barkeep. Again he saw the day he had come home from school and Mutt, his mongrel love, had been so glad to see him that he'd broken the tip of his tail on the newel as he came charging downstairs, wildly a-wag. The splint, which embarrassed the dog, was a dangerous weapon when Mutt thrashed out his greetings.

Puttering around in this dusty memory-shed, the young man recalled the first job he ever had. After school he had gone to work for the ZCMI. The Zion Cooperative Mercantile Institute, an elegant department store, allowed him to earn enough money to buy six magnificent teaspoons, artistically decorated with bunched grapes on their handles, and housed in a sateen-lined purple box. It was a kingly gift and his stepmother lavished praise that trembled him with joy.

It would soon be time for the train. He bought his seventh Scotch, watched a customer pour half a dozen silver dollars into the big fortune wheel without a win, and lighted another Piedmont. The smoke pulled him back to Olivet Hospital. Shame for his behavior at his father's bedside made him blush. He wiped the fresh-sprung moisture from his forehead and, of all the things he might have remembered about his father, one of the jokes he used to say was dominant. A wry quirk in the young man's nature made him say the line aloud.

"I'm as tickled right now as if I'd run a nail in my foot."

CHAPTER 14

He that is used to go forward and findeth a stop, falleth out of his own favor, and is not the thing he was.—Francis Bacon

LIKE the pattern set by his disease, the sick man's spirits rose and fell during the early months of his restriction to his room. Happily the great weight was on the up side. There were one or two prolonged depressive periods but most of the glooms were come-and-go and not all that hard to rassle to the floor.

At one time, when his progress was so much slower than his predecessor guinea pigs' progress had been, he fretted himself into braking his recovery. How it goes in the mind makes how the body goes. Nailed to the bed, each day outdragged the next. It was a struggle for him to crawl up out of the barrel without feeling sorry enough for himself to bring on the upchucks. His guardian cherub must have enjoined him to pull his socks up.

"So time does clomp along in lead sneakers," his seraphic buddy said. "There'll be a lot more drag than that unless you sprinkle your blues with a little hope-dust."

A poet once said that not everyone is tuned to the same tambourine. Time can go as treacle flows or speed at a panic pace. Time moves in keeping with the severity of the maladies, leavened by the disposition of the ailing. Sick time is slower than well time. And depressive thinking is natural to the ill.

It came on the myasthenic, in this mood, with a kind of

weary sorrow, that we die a little when we fail our firm resolves. A part of innocence is lost and there is no scapegoat to take us off the hook. These defeats are in ourselves. They are not in the compulsions of the world, however we fiddle the truth.

Each of the failures added to man's burden in the Mazda-Ahriman conflict, in which evil's assaults have been, long, long before recorded history, more potent than the overweening good.

When the righteous man's wrath prevails and he thrashes the foe, unlike that enemy, he rests from the fray and turns his hand to more agreeable pursuits. The evil forces have been bruised and reduced. But they persist. And it is in this perpetuation that they differ so markedly from the good men. Evil is a purity. Unhappily there is a dilution in good men and true. Natural goodness does not extend to the bottom of the human heart.

In his forced state of discomfort, such depressive thoughts came down on the myasthenic like the wolf on the fold. He was crowded, too, by practical misgivings. The economic future was bleak. How was he going to infuse his anemic bank account against the day he and his wife would have to look after a couple of old people whose income wasn't big enough to take care of them?

A major fear was that he might live too long.

His public-relations business, which had shown fair promise, had been guillotined the year before by his London crisis. Since then he'd been too ill to work. The longer he was out of circulation, the more business contacts would wither. Contacts in his line of work were as essential as clients. On top of that he was sure that his contemporaries regarded him, understandably, as too unreliable to tie into. He wasn't a young man any more and he was obviously severely ill.

A few hours later, or it might have been sooner, this vexatious maundering hit bottom. The very weight of the depressive tea party levered up a kind of bravado to stiffen the psychic jelly. Like the time he tried to make a joke on the stretcher outside an operating room, waiting to be wheeled in. Dopey from the injection they'd given him in the ward, he wasn't able to muster more than a whisper for the waiting anesthetist.

"Do me a favor?" he asked the big blonde.

"If I can." They were always so noncommittal.

"Don't let them sew me up with red thread. I prefer plaid. Not so ostentatious."

She gave him a dutiful laugh. It made him feel better. Sometimes whistling as you pass the cemetery stones is good music. If things went wrong in the cut-up room, any pre-operative fee-blings would be sheer waste. If a fellow has to spend at such a time, the best thing is to squander. There was some nervous comfort in that notion.

When both sides of the column had been added up for these wearying weeks, there had been despond but no despair. For when the bale was just this side of too heavy to lift, the sweet juices would flow up from that well he had never measured but which he knew was deep enough. Let the psychic darts be hurled with whatever force. The human will has the power to fortify the walls.

Part of the problem of being obliged to stumble through an alien land is in the knowing that dangers abound. Some can be spotted in time to bob and weave. And that's a comfort. But it is no secret that there are land mines and booby traps that will be discovered only when they are stepped on or prodded.

As the trees thin out, it gets easier to see which way is best to travel. Much of the jungle fear fades. And then it is possible to sort out the perilous journey, remembering the twistings and turnings that came up okay, carefully noting those that had dire consequences. On such intelligence, sound warnings can be raised to warn the travelers yet to come. The sick man felt a strong obligation to leave a useful striggle.

There is an aloneness on such journeys in spite of all the people who rally round. These troubled feelings are intensified with age. A sick man is a sicker man when he has long passed his prime and is way down the catabolic slope.

Yet, as he plowed this field, sitting in his room with no distractions, he was convinced that strong purpose and determination form the best defense against the threat of defeat. Whenever he would fail in this resolve he would beat himself and send the bucket down into the well again, vowing to be stronger on the next go-round.

There were of course relapses from those resurrections. One early evening in June, flaked out by the strain of a long bout of suctioning, a ruptured trach-tube cuff, and the discomfort of having a new tube jammed into the stoma, he was bathed in melancholy vapors. Repeatedly he prodded the call button for attention he didn't need and normally wouldn't have asked for. With customary patience, the nurses fielded his frets.

97

And then something happened. What flipped the switch, he'd never know. Some star in the cosmos exploded and it came all clear to him what was happening. He was becoming a professional patient! He was becoming the sick body that *more* than accepts what is being done for it. He was demanding this attention as his due, as what he was entitled to by the very act of being ill, and by its sister act, just being there. He could hear himself bellowing his demands.

Cure me, doctor!

Tend me, nurse!

I will lie here on my bed of pain and suffering (there is melancholy music soft in the background here) and you must make me well again. That is, if you can. And I ain't all that sure that you can manage it, either.

Pull up, old son. You're riding the brake pedal. You're on the road that leads to enjoyment of poor health, a road as dangerous as it is soppy.

The patient must join the others in trying to help the patient.

Common sense insists that mental attitudes can slow or speed the healing processes. Warmth and affection, too. From both sides of the street.

Warmed by the glow of his optimistic sermon, he saw himself thundering at the world of the downbeat to pull up their dressings and get actively into the act.

These fulminations did more than comfort the man. His disposition demanded periodic drama. He was a ham. And dear-bought experience had long since convinced him that it was error to rely only on the high beat of excitement, the adrenal peaks, to carry the day. There comes a time when, no matter what, it all seems downhill. For these Sisyphean days strong resolution must be invoked. Audacity, too. He had never seen it as seemly to make too modest demands of life. Daring, unless the individual character rejects audacity as the body might refuse transplanted organs, is what is wanted at such times. Not mad, idiot derring-do. Not rash valor. Sensible audacity. More battles are won with sensible audacity than are lost.

Go lightly on the debates. Refrain from demand for studied solutions. There are times when it is wisdom to let the gut take over. Feel. Become indignant. Raise a raging clamor against the illness and the constrictions it imposes. Make waves. Rock boats.

Cry out against the lowering of the curtain. Go center stage and declaim defiance.

In a short while, unless there is a pie audience, this expression of high resolve might get as hollow as a fallen log. But worth its while, if you haven't lost your sense of humor.

He didn't think he had.

Of course it isn't always easy for the seriously ill to be rational. Pressure and strain, man's constant companions through this vale, are his bitterest enemies, sick or well. They churn the digestive tract of the healthiest man. They are murder to the myasthenic. Fears and resentments turn quickly into impotence. Anger and anxiety shorten the wind, make chest pains, send some of the corpuscles skittering around like frightened mice, and tamper with the operation of the glands.

At such times it is only natural to look to the doctor to make it all well. But cure doesn't come on demand. The patient's failure to see that *he* must do a big part of the job means he is looking through the wrong end of the glass. That's when it's time to ease off; to come up gentle on the complaints; to hold the line. *Ils ne passeront pas!* Which reminded him he'd have to do some homework on those French verbs.

Most of the time the myasthenic was mulish on the bitter end. Hang in there, whatever the contest, until it was irrevocably decided. How many times, he reminded himself, had he played pool at The Players and seen the eight ball hanging on the lip of the pocket. Put it down and you're a hero. It's as easy as a three-inch putt.

But the over-confident pool-shooter's aim on that cinch-shot can be hurried or careless. He aims. He shoots. He flubs it! The cue ball, struck badly, catches the corner of the pocket and nudges the eight ball an inch or two along the rail. Not into the pocket. Along the rail.

To every ear but his own, the self-victim's scream of agony is fully symphonic. Oh, it is music to the gambler's ears to hear the sucker squeal. It is never over until the eight ball is deep down in that pocket.

Do not concede. Never resign.

Once, he would sadly recall, when he was on the Hollywood High School track team, he had eased up just a few feet from the tape in the 880, confident he had the race. But the lad right behind him, with an adrenal burst, hit the string first. That loss bothered the Connecticut myasthenic most of his adult life. It had something to do with the intensity of his conviction that up-giving is not a desirable exercise.

Now that the clutch of depressive clouds had cleared, the sick man's sky was brightened further by the progress reports of the first two myasthenics who had been treated with the predni-sone therapy.

Number one, a slight and wiry man of forty-five or so, had responded from the very outset to the high single-dose, alter-nate-day oral regimen. In the first three days that followed the initial dose of the drug, his strength and stamina increased and the symptoms markedly diminished. On the fifteenth day he did so well the doctors were surprised. By the fiftieth, he was well enough to pack up the old kit bag and go on home. Gossip on the ward had it that he went right back to work and walked five miles a day. Mailman, likely.

Number two was a fifty-five-year-old woman who had come out of her tunnel in three months' time. Her case had been a bit more stubborn than number one's but not as stubborn as number three's. Not that she'd had an easy time of it. She had started from a rugged base. Eight years of peaks and valleys in general strength, deterioration of facial, chewing, and swallowing mus-cles, cosmetic problems, and fluctuating voice weakness. Mestinon and several other anticholinesterase drugs delivered lessening ben-efits. She was in a bad way when she arrived at the Clinical Cen-ter.

She responded well but slowly to the therapy, but toward the end of her hundred days on the drug, just when it looked like she was on the verge of swallowing success, she aspirated fluid in her windpipe. Floundered around like a carp out of water until orderly breathing had been restored. She was furious at these set-backs, impatient with the snail's trot of the therapy. She would pace her room in smouldering frustration, like big cats do in the zoos. But she was a determined female and although she hadn't all those options that were hers before the swallowing muscles re-treated, she came back to the battleground full of fight after each of her seismic skirmishes.

The therapy, backstopped by her determination, paid off handsomely. She walked out of the hospital, head high.

With her husband, she devoted time to the local myasthenia

gravis group, and when she returned to the Clinical Center for checkups, she'd stop in on every myasthenic on the ward to try to lift languid spirits. She was living proof of how well the dread disease could be contained.

She was a natural visitor. An easy talker. Assembled in any one of the rooms, they combed the benefits to be expected from different drugs and dosages, and whether silver trach-tubes were more comfortable than plastic. There was much talk about weight, which she was putting on, now that she could swallow, and about which she clucked disapprovingly. She loved good food. Abstention had been a torment. Besides, steroids increase body weight, which boosts the rigorous demands of dieting. Yet even this could not deflate her bubbling happiness at no more danger of sucking food and drink into her lungs.

Aspiration is major evidence of feeble muscles. Minor manifestations can be important, too. When the myasthenic is bound to his bed by muscles too weak to work, there is ample time to reflect on such simple acts as raising an eyebrow, licking a lip, blowing a Bronx cheer (or a raspberry, if preference dictates), making a moue. How important to screw the face into these gestures. So important, when they can't be practiced. And no intricate machinery is involved. All the more frustrating when, with all the power of concentrated will, he could not conjure up a single one of them.

He sulked. Not long. The dour mood passed, as others had before it. He was helped on the way by attention to his calculation of his target dates. It was a heady supposition, but what if the beneficial effects of the prednisone were cumulative and he enjoyed a sharp improvement, as guinea pig number one had done? There wasn't much chance this dream would come true, but if it did—he would be in the cat-bird seat around May the twentieth. Failing to grab this brass ring, it could be the middle of June when hallelujahs could be lofted to heaven. Middle of June would make it about three months since he started on the prednisone. Three months was number two's time.

He accepted that this hope could die a-borning, too. But by now he was better prepared for disappointment. When he and his Greenwich neurologist had first talked about the NIH program he had somehow believed that the curative period of prednisone would be no longer than the ACTH course—three weeks or so, at most.

By disposition he was a hasty and impatient man. Always

had been. It was an ego trait that was to plague him all his days. On rare occasions the bright light would flash on and he would plainly see Wishful Thinking transmogrified into Broken Promise.

However such situations went, they had to be dealt with. What it seemed to boil down to was that he'd better try to stay fairly comfortable and not fret himself, so's the magic chemical could do its stuff. *Pas de se tracasser,* as a Frenchman might put it. His Larousse said it meant not to fuss or worry or fret or vex. Not bad for a motto.

Of course, it wasn't all that easy. It never is, he told himself wryly, just sitting there, fretting a little in spite of Larousse.

This was a time when no amount of will would move a single muscle and when diversions would fail to divert. He sat in a puddle of guilt because he wasn't handling his indisposition properly and he wasn't making anything out of the time he was trying to kill. Never mind what. He could have been cramming his irregular French verbs or plotting a story for when he would be able to write again. But pinned down by the respirator's umbilical, he just wasn't perking any too well. Lethargic. Once or twice he crawled into small dark pockets of disquiet. And once he went deep enough to string himself out so tight he would have howled at the top of his lungs to relieve the tension, if only his voice box would work. Since he couldn't make even a mouse-squeak, he was impelled all the more to bellow his frustrations. Rubber bands, he told himself sententiously, can be stretched just so far. (At times he was inclined to puny aphorisms.) But he was finally getting to be an old hand at tensions and knew better now how to handle them. There would probably have been no yelling at all, even if he had had his voice. There certainly would not have been a repeat of the Battle of the Bell, his blowup in the hospital in Manhattan when he was tapering off a rugged course of ACTH. He was still disgusted with himself for that shocking lack of self-control. Probably one of the sorriest questions we ever ask ourselves is "Why did I do *that?*"

He had learned something from that sorry exhibition. The vital importance of self-control, no matter the circumstances, for one. And a little more patience. Patience had never been one of his crowning glories. But he was not completely unarmed to grapple with this failing. A sense of the ridiculous can be a sharp sword. As on the day he sucked custard into his windpipe, trying to eat without benefit of the tube in his nose. It was almost worth the torment of the aspiration. After the outraged trachea had been cleared and he had his breath back, he was gripped by an unreasonable fury that the swallowing muscles had failed again, just when it looked like he had cleared the hurdle.

Balls! Balls to it!

And the very moment his mind had framed the word he was engulfed in a belly laugh of heavenly proportions.

Of all the associations he might have made with that Anglo-Saxon malediction, why had such a singular connection as an ancient doggerel been made? He hadn't heard the verse for donkey's years but the word had called it forth.

> *It was Christmas in the harem*
> *And the eunuchs all were there,*
> *Watching the lovely maidens*
> *Comb their lustrous hair,*
> *When suddenly the sultan's voice*
> *Resounded through the halls,*
> *"What'll you have for Christmas, boys?"*
> *And the eunuchs answered, "Balls."*

The laughter made him feel much better, though it would have been more fun to share it. The incident demonstrated that there are all manner of ways to wipe out the up-tight fantods. Over the distance, though, the most satisfying defenses against these inner storms were the mental excursions: picking over bits and pieces of philosophy, nosing into books or tuning the good music stations, emulating Marcel Proust, that eccentric Frenchman who spent his declining ten years in an unventilated bedroom calling up the past.

CHAPTER 15

◄§ *Memory gathers roses in winter.*

His room was unusually active in the mornings. Medication, vital signs, hand-tests, respirometer trials, bath, bed-make, cleanup. Busy. The rest of the day came on kind of quiet. At night, before lights out, he was on his own.

Eyes closed, relaxed, it was a good time to thumb the pages of his life and rediscover passages of power and beauty that had shaped and molded him. Sometimes there would be relevance to his illness in the memories. Sometimes, weeks or months later, when he recalled them, he would make the association himself. In any case, as he churned up the past, the reruns would come on with crystal clarity.

Like the time years ago when he was working on the *Los Angeles Times*, doing moonlight movie jobs, writing a column for a Chicago paper, and running all over town without half enough sleep. When the chance came along to get away from the rat race for a while, he grabbed it. One of the boys in the city room wanted to switch vacation periods, so he took his two weeks early, drove up into the Owens Valley to a town called Independence, just north of Mt. Whitney.

He rented a fiery, wiry piebald to carry him into the mountains. On introduction in the corral they eyed each other speculatively. One, approvingly; the other, with dubiety. A half-hearted attempt to toss the city gent had been made when he climbed aboard. He had been expecting some such dido. It had not been difficult to make clear who was going to do what to whom. From then on they were in love.

It hadn't taken long for the liveryman to convince his customer that he'd need a packhorse for the length of the proposed camp-out and the gear he was planning to take. A lot of stuff that's never used is hauled up and back on mountain trips. His overpack may have been urged by all those Westerns, where the arc-legged hero forks his faithful cayuse, rides out yonder into gawd's country fer months on end with no more'n the trusty carbine, a cuttin' knife, and a brace of tiddly saddlebags. The movies are the movies. This here was mountain country. Packhorse, welcome aboard.

Now, in his mind's eye, as clear as the day it had happened nearly forty years before, the sick man saw himself, young and strong and filled with the lust of living, headed west toward Kearsarge Pass, up through the sparsely settled first shelf of the towering Sierra. The twisting road, soon shrinking itself into narrowing trails as it climbed, led out of the green valley toward the Bull Frog Lakes district, where he was to set up camp. At that time of the year the lakes were always loaded with mottled and speckled beauties, but the lakes' remoteness discouraged all but the most devoted anglers.

Several times on their way up the side of the mountain they would come onto stretches of fairly level road that ran on for respectable distances. The horse, happy to be free of stable boredom, would prance and caper to persuade his rider to increase the pace. Too bad that stodgy packhorse had to be tagging along. The piebald and his rider did find a stretch to indulge in a blood-stirring spurt of speed, but it wasn't the time or the place to let the vigorous mount run free. Once over the pass, lake-side, they would drop the gear and hobble the pack animal. There'd be plenty of room there to run together, as much as it pleasured them.

In the picture on the memory screen, he saw himself nearing the top of the east slope of the high cut, just before taking the sharp turn that would ease through the notch and onto the lakes. Slowly they were skirting a deep, shale-sided sink, a huge, inverted cone, with a snow-rimmed pool of black-blue water a hundred yards below the trail. The snows sharpened the vistas in every direction and the soul-washing process was well under way. There was always snow that high in the Sierra in July. It sharpened the water in the pit to a deeper, stronger blue than the bright sky of that cloudless day. Now and then rock fragments and bits of shale would loosen and go slithering down to plop and plunk into the icy tarn.

Looking down, the rider was not too comfortable. Here the trail was at its narrowest. He pressed his leg tighter against the side of the horse that seemed literally to hang over the lip of the chasm. It was the same unconscious demand that used to make passengers lean away from the low wing of a sharply banking airplane. A fall off that mountain path would be as final as any fall out of the sky. Once over the edge of the narrow trail, down the scarp and into the water, neither he nor the horse would ever find footing enough to scramble to safety.

In a way, it was like that in the hospital room in Bethesda. Critically ill, he may well have seen himself sliding the steep sides of a hole he might not be able to climb out of. More likely it had been sometime later that he'd made the parallel association between his plight and that day in the Sierra.

For the next several waning hours, mnemonic pictures, larded with dozing and spurts of sickroom attention, crowded onto the screen. Their distractions were fleeting. He was tired. It had been a long day. His mind was skittering around like a leaf along a windy lane.

The nurse, hearing the bubbling splutter of the fluids that were building up in his windpipe, flipped her hands expertly into rubber gloves, cleared the catheter from its antiseptic envelope in an easy, sweeping motion, fitted the fluted end of the thin rubber tube into the air-hose, pushed it gently into the trachea, sucked out the secretions, and made him comfortable again. He eased off, in a kind of small exhaustion, and fell sound asleep.

In the days ahead, when he took those excursions into the past, it wasn't memory exactly. Sometimes it was more of a mental *feeling*, a sensory review of bits and pieces of himself, frequently out of any semblance of continuity. Divergent scenes would run into each other in mad disregard of sensible association. It would seem as if he sensed rather than remembered deep convictions of his youth, why he had embraced them and what they had meant to him.

Was it possible, he would wonder on more than one occasion, that his disease could bear upon his psyche or his intellect as well as upon his body?

Before he had been so severely stricken, when he had gone

into his past, it was usually on demand for data bearing on a current problem. Black-and-white recall. He remembered or he didn't. No foggy musings. No mist or ghostly maybes. And failure to peg his recollections to accurate calendar dates rarely mattered very much. But now, when he failed to sharpen the focus, his anamnestic adventures came only partially alive. Recall was either not enough or much too much; too tender, as the flesh is tender under abraded skin.

The perplexities of indecision often extended themselves into worry. Concern would likely be a better word.

This myasthenia-crippled man was nearly seventy years old. He'd spent more time on earth than most men attain, even in these days of high life expectancy. How had he used his three score and ten? How had he spent such a generous sum?

Whatever review was to be undertaken, more was called for than a cursory series of flashes, like those one is supposed to experience before going down for the third time. Instead, the sick man felt an almost desperate need for a quiet recall of the values he had determined in his long life. There is no better time, he could not have been more certain, to ponder these values, these criteria one has lived with and by, than when life is threatened.

Almost as if the words were being flashed onto the electric news-ribbon that wound itself around that building on the Times Square island in Manhattan, he saw the question sharp and clear.

Of all that I have known and done in my full years, what do I prize most and what would I miss most bitterly?

He leaned back against the pillows, closed his eyes, and walked gently into the clock as is done in dreams, unencumbered by reality. Only in this way could he see all that was crowded onto his plate. And the major events are by no means the only milestones. Each man is the sum of all that he has touched and that has touched him, even so slight as a passing glance.

But only so much territory can be explored. Only so much can be withdrawn from that unbelievably copious warder of the brain, that storehouse of everything.

Which of all his touchings used to matter most? And which of them matter now? Of all the events and occurrences, what display could be chosen by this ailing bag of bones to hang upon the wall, without too abject apology, as his epitaph?

He had earned a fair living in a variety of ways, mostly with a typewriter. Now and again his work had given more pleasure than the paycheck showed. Sometimes he had kicked pebbles out of less happy paths. He'd met a mess of people and dealt with them in divers ways, as they had dealt with him. Too often he had behaved selfishly but now and again had spent himself on others for their own sakes. He had thoroughly enjoyed most of what had befallen him and had always delighted in being alive. One thing for double sure: he had wasted vastly too much time.

There was no bonanza for posterity in this thumbnail. His earthly passage would not be marked, alas, by a splendid symphony, fine writing, great ideas, or good works. But he had never wanted for adventure and excitement and beauty to remember. And love. He had had a very fair share.

No mean adventure was the great fall from the cliff he was trying to scale when he'd run away from school in Mobile. He was young for a mountaineer and the scarp was formidable. At not yet eight, ten feet straight up is high. There were no broken bones, although he squealed like a stuck pig when he thumped onto his rump.

Other pictures out of the past welled up with artesian force. There was the perpetual-motion machine he had invented just after his father and Jessie and he had moved to Los Angeles in the middle teens and had taken the white frame house off Maple Avenue.

Dr. Robert Millikan had asked to see the machine called mechanically impossible that had sprung from the schoolboy's mind. How contact had been made with one of the world's most eminent scientists, he could not remember now. A letter, perhaps, written to the California Institute of Technology, the most likely nearby place where there might be interest in such a device, may have come to the physicist's eye. This learned man, who was to receive a Nobel award a few years later, could have persuaded himself to test and perhaps to encourage an acquisitive young mind that had chosen to leap over the massive bulk of the world's physical problems to subdue a monster. It might just as well have been that Dr. Millikan was a wise and kindly man, with an ample buttering of curiosity and a need for odd diversion. In any case, an invitation to demonstrate the perpetual-motion machine had been extended and the boy could hardly tie the string, he was that excited, as he packed his dream in a stout box and carried it on the long trolley ride to Pasadena.

In this version of the perpetual-motion machine, more than a dozen cord-thin glass tubes, which had cost him many mowed lawns, were held securely around the rim of a small glass funnel with adhesive tape. They were shaped like tiny canes, with their lower ends extended into a large bowl from which water would be sucked upward by capillary attraction, to discharge the water, drop by drop, into the funnel. The tubes would provide enough water to turn the little waterwheel affixed to the end of the spout. It would then fall back into the reservoir, whence the process would be repeated over and over and over. A never-ending cycle, as could plainly be seen. Perpetual motion. Energy generated out of itself.

The boy was proudly excited as he demonstrated the machine and the little waterhweel turned slowly round and round. The famous scientist praised him for his imagination and ingenuity. Then, in a gentle way, he explained why the device would fail. Even as he spoke, the little wheel began to slow. Soon it would stop. They didn't have long to wait.

The villain was surface tension. Friction dragged at the water in the thread-thin tubes and the rising columns of liquid were no longer strong enough to break through the convex beads that formed on the end of each tube and clung tenaciously.

Once again the answer to this ancient problem remained to be revealed. But the boy's failure was not the tragedy it could have been. The worldly doctor had managed the drama so skillfully that the boy went away warmed almost to a glow by the adventure. The praise and the attention he'd been given was far more than disappointment could dispel.

The mind is indeed an antic instrument. With vivid clarity, in infinite detail, and with miraculous speed, he relived dozens of years of his life, perhaps as fully in review as when the events actually occurred.

It was surprising how fully those early days—the middle teens—unfolded on his memory screen. Those were the days in Los Angeles when bungalows and stucco boxes had orange groves as neighbors; when the growing city had not yet turned west toward the Pacific and there were acres and acres of open ground, some of it set out to flowers and vegetables, just beyond Westlake Park.

Pepper trees shaded the back-lot of Famous Players-Lasky (later to become Paramount) at Sunset and Vine, where he would get his first job in the movies. An office boy. Once again in his mind he saw, from a blistered window of his apartment, the towering flames eat up most of Warner Brothers studio on Sunset Boulevard.

There were love affairs with three famous movie stars, respectfully spaced in time, to be sure. One of these engagements was outstandingly memorable. It was not easy to couple, on a sunny California hillside, while the horses browsed contentedly nearby, when she was in jodhpurs and he was in breeches and boots.

There was a hummingbird who returned day after day to hang at the fringe of the heady honeysuckle. Surf-swimming at the beach house at Malibu. And grunion hunts in moonlight. Riding an eager palomino on an early winter morning along the north shore of Lake Arrowhead, just before the season's first fall of snow.

It was the peak of elation to see the Eiffel Tower poking its iron finger through the early evening haze as the Super-Constellation came in off the Channel and followed the Seine to Le Bourget. And the exquisite gut-pang, muscles knotted into a searing ball, as he plunged, nose down, in a Black Widow nightfighter at six hundred miles an hour.

The Wednesday night, in the Press Club poker game, when his pair of fours outbluffed aces-up to haul in the night's biggest pot. And the mummy they dug up, looking very little like mummies he'd seen in museums, at the base of the step pyramid at Saqqara, on the Nile. Never mind he was a man in his forties. He quivered like a schoolgirl at her first prom to be standing at the oldest man-made structure in the world. It did something for his soul to ponder the past in Rome's Colosseum at midnight, with hundreds of cats for company instead of lions. And leaning forward so as not to miss a single syllable the day Winston Churchill crossed words with Aneurin Bevan in the House of Commons.

Now the recollections were tailgating themselves. He was reading *Jean Christophe* for the first time. Tuning in the New York Philharmonic on an old Atwater Kent radio. Launching rude and raucous choruses of "Three Old Ladies Locked In The Lava'try" across the Thames from the Prospect of Whitby's balcony. Gingerly biting into a sheep's eye at an Arab feast in a date grove just outside Manama in Bahrein. Singing a song. Tickling a trout. Discovering anything. Being.

Never mind up-and-doing all the time. Just being was enough. Like the animals men insist are lesser. Keeping an eye out for enemies and food. But most of the time, being.

If he ticked off a thousand more delights, he wouldn't begin

111

to list the wonderful things the world is crowded with. There are more than enough miseries, true. But this is the only world in the neighborhood. It was his disposition to bend toward the compensations.

Gingerly he stepped out of this brain-bath to reflect on the spiritual convictions that were essential to his life. He held irrevocably that each man is responsible for what he does, and should be held to that account. He was not inclined to word-flog the proposition. That a child's parents fail in their obligations to instill the virtues of responsibility in their offspring is indeed a wicked burden on the little animal. And more's the pity. But such omission does not absolve abominable behavior.

Pride may indeed be the deadliest of the seven sins, but it is not man's most wicked effort. Early in his San Francisco days he had been profoundly moved by the works of an Austrian novelist. He never pulled another trigger.

Killing is not sport.

The proselyte's pressure to bow to his gods as the true and only gods is an abomination.

Hypocrisy is disgusting.

Cruelty is a massive sin.

Timon's words tell the painful truth: The unkindest beast is kinder than mankind.

As long ago as his teens, the myasthenic had made judgments on such crochets as superstition, which he thought was more ridiculous than wicked, if torch and stake were not involved. Unlike astrology and her sister pseudos, this low-slung discipline is seldom taken lightly enough to be amusing.

Metaphysics, which someone once said is wrangling over things needless to be known, was not his cup of tea, although people he cared a great deal about had found it satisfying. A thing like this can be a dancy bar. A judgment formed for those he loved, by those he loved. What-ho the values of the "ology." A scholar he was not. Nor a preacher. After a three-pack-a-day renunciation he certainly didn't hold with smoking, but he couldn't see any sense in snatching idiot-sticks out of the mouths of the misguided to prove his point.

How he believed was how he himself believed. And none was called upon to join him. Each man must file his own flight plan. And each man can. For we do what we want to do, if the doing can be done. The targets we raise in the butts—and the bull's eyes, near-misses, and bloops—are the products of our own humors, dispositions, and environments.

Twisting in this narrow box, the myasthenic once again asked himself why he took the turnings he knew he didn't want to take. And yet he had taken them. What spurs us to these sad decisions? Motives are lurky beasts, averse so frequently to showing themselves enough to be identified with accuracy. Too often definitions that do not define are made, accepted, and acted on with the fervor of Holy Church. Sight and judgment are too often hasty and scampered.

So thinking, it occurred to the sick man that there are benefits in a serious illness, presuming one outlives it. For openers, there are fewer imperatives in the course of daily living. This provides time to try on new ideas, aberrant or otherwise, for size.

Sloshing these notions around on his mental tongue suggested that this is one of man's major problems. He doesn't have the time or inclination to climb into the sky often enough. He's prone to go along too many times, when it would be better all around to lay down at least one roadblock. Fail to shoot the moon, at least once in a while, and a man will never savor one of life's most delicious flavors. Like winning a race everybody but the runner knows is lost. Or outguessing vaunted experts. Or lending money to a man who pays it back, long after they all knew he would welsh the debt.

These are not cerebral matters. They must be gut-felt. For, when the chips are down and the log is split and all those other allegorical clichés are piped over the side, when it is known out of the head instead of the loins or the heart, it is likely to be more often wrong than right.

Sometimes, when the invalid was dancing through these raindrops, he had sense enough not to take himself too seriously. Happily this touch of sanity was present when he felt inclined to complain at the length of time it was taking his magic medicine to improve his circumstances. He just didn't seem to be getting anywhere. Plateau. He wanted action. Understandable. Especially since most people are conditioned to expect sharp and rapid response to the medicines they are given. Commercials on the cyclops, a pet aversion, had made a heavy contribution to this fiction.

He was by now too seasoned to expect immediate recovery of muscle strength, but he did feel it was about time for a change.

A little better luck than plateau-stalling. He put great stock in chance. He was sure about chance, that unsurest of all phenomena. Chance is a chameleon. It is the good luck some people call prosperity. And the bad luck they label adversity. Only one thing is sure about chance: luck will always change. An eminently fair proposition, in his book.

Chance is a field wide enough to be lighthearted and capersome in. As when there is a high wager on which sugar lump the fly will see as a landing strip. Or a disquisition on why "heads" or "tails" is called when a coin is flipped. Never in the singular. Well, hardly ever. And chance is a very narrow field where blade to jugular is the only answer when the bangtail, toting the family fortune, chases his trackmates all the way home.

Somewhere between Messrs. Scylla and Charybdis, an ailing man can almost enjoy himself reckoning up the odds on his recovery chances. And to speculate on the possibility of optimistic resolution having power enough to sway the inequalities of happenstance.

There was no one time the Clinical Center inmate was more basically optimistic than another. Even when he was bed-bound and tied to the breathing-machine he was more often than not sure he'd come out of it. And when he could make it out of bed and into the easy chair, even with a little help, and from there to the bathroom and back, his surety increased. Staggerings and wobblings were the order of the day. But it was on his own, and that made him swinging a fair go. Fair enough to make it an odds-on bet, in spite of the London trouble, the surgery, the brittle periods, and all.

CHAPTER 16

*A hundred-load of worry will not pay
an ounce of debt.—Jacula Prudentum*

A vaudeville team, whose names have been wiped from memory by time, had played the Orpheum Theater in Los Angeles in the early twenties. They dressed as World War doughboys and they did their act in a set that suggested the trenches. The soppy one, grotesque in a strangulating uniform, could have been Stan Laurel's twin brother. He was scared witless. In character he was a naturally funny man and used a piece of running business that never failed to pull laughter from deep in the audience-belly.

At each report in the steady, offstage cannonading that simulated shelling the very trench he was crouched in, he would jerk in terror enough to tilt the undersized tin hat that was perched atop his steel-wool hair, blinding him. The groping hand he sent up to find the helmet's rim to lift it and clear his eyes never seemed to find the mark without protracted fumbling. Sometimes this idiotic search went on for minutes, as he milked his audience as only an artist can. And then he would screw his face up, whimper in falsetto, and weep in abject, comic fright.

The funny man's eupeptic buddy would try to sweet-reason him out of his funk.

"Ca'mon now, pal. Pull ya'self together. Whatcha worried about? On'y two things can happen to ya. Either ya gonna get hit or ya ain't gonna get hit. If ya ain't hit, there ain't nuthin' ta worry about. If ya do get hit, on'y two things can happen to ya. Either it's gonna be a scratch or it's gonna be bad. If it's a scratch, what's to care? An' if it's a bad one, on'y two things can happen. Ya gonna get well or ya ain't gonna get well. If ya do get well, you ain't got nuthin' ta worry about. An' if ya *don't* get well—old buddy, ya sure ain't gonna be able ta worry. So why worry?"

CHAPTER 17

Life is one long tragedy.—W. Winwood Reade
Life is sweet.—English proverb

ONE day, early in June, they wheeled in a new Bennett respirator. Latest model. Bigger. More sophisticated, as they say, than the machine he'd been on for weeks. It was smoother in operation than the Bird breathing-machine that was now relegated to standby. Despite its size the new Bennett had fewer knobs and dials than any of its predecessors. Easier for him to control the flow and rhythm of the air-intake. Same old story: whatever it is, if you make it simpler, you make it better.

Regardless of what kind of respirator was in use, one thing remained unchanged. Artificial respiration means suctioning. Secretions that dormant throat muscles couldn't handle had to be pulled out of the trachea and bronchial tubes many times a day. Normally these body fluids move down the pharynx through the esophagus into the stomach. When the swallowing muscles are on holiday, as with myasthenia, the opening into the trachea is not closed off and the secretions flow down the windpipe. If enough accumulate, damned if a man can't drown in his own juices. Literally.

Care had always to be taken to prevent infection, because the catheters are threaded through the tracheostomy-tube directly into the weasand, which is what Mr. Shakespeare calls the windpipe. Most of the Clinical Center nurses were deft at suctioning and disposed of the liquids quickly and easily. A few had a tendency to stab and probe with the catheter as they went deep into the bronchi to pick up all the offending juices. This got the job done adequately, most times. Not always thoroughly. Never comfortably.

Suctioning can be a psychological as well as a physical proposition. It is vexatious to be forced to realize that life can be threatened by one's own secretions and that a man is at the mercy of a rubber straw stuck through a hole in his throat.

The stretch of days that were all of a stamp continued to try his patience. The doctors would come into his room periodically, make the usual muscle-reaction tests, and talk about the long, slow curve on the chart rising. Rising slowly, perhaps, but rising. A very good sign. The doctors were pleased at the progress, but the patient, try as he would, didn't feel any upswings taking place. He found it increasingly difficult to see the progress the doctors said they saw. The sick man believed they might be giving him verbal placebos. Nonetheless, one way or another he'd get through the waking hours after the doctors had gone. It was when the day had been buttoned up and sleep seemed remote as the Cape of Good Hope that he most hated his prison.

In the quiet of his room, ruffled only by the murmur of the respirator, a parade of cosmic problems would begin to assemble. The range was far from mingy. Sometimes it was a search for the solution to a mate-in-two chess problem; sometimes the problems were more serious than chess. Like, where is the point at which the human life should no longer be sustained?

Out of all the time and thoughtful attention he paid to this question, it came down to no more than that old Numerian proverb. It depends on whose ox is being gored.

For the myasthenic, if the body in the sickbed is a vegetable, death is a coveted prize. His own illness reinforced this view. But how the other fellow might want to handle it—that was up to him.

Of course he didn't spend all of his sleep-wooing on such lofty arcanae. Most of the time, to serve the truth, he let his mind meander. And that passes the time, too.

Then, one April day, it happened!
His chest muscles stirred!
Were they really coming alive? It was time to find out. And

so he reached up and disengaged the rubber band that held the air hose nipple securely in place in his trach-tube. He opened the hemostat and collapsed the cuff. There weren't too many secretions. So he plugged the hole in the trach-tube and began to breathe. On his own!

The air came in and the air went out. Feebly. But in and out. And after a very little time the intercostals tired and he had to plug himself back into the respirator.

He was bathed in a joyful wave. Difficult to restrain himself. He wanted to cut out the breathing-machine and try it on his own again. Right now. But he knew that the chest muscles had to be rested. So he counted out five minutes by his watch. Then he unplugged himself again and did some more breathing under his own power. Again only feeble inhalations. But still on his own. That was what counted.

His fingers trembled as he punched the call-bell button. The nurses were as happy as he was. So were the doctors. It had taken quite a while.

Now it was off the Bennett for longer and longer periods. These performances were paced. He had to take it easy. It wouldn't do to press the awakening muscles too heavily. Next day he went off the machine for five full minutes. Then ten. Then thirty. An hour. Five. And it was done!

April was a big month that year. They turned off the artificial respirator and never turned it on again for him. For days he savored April 22, as one does a treasured anniversary, reliving again and again the stirrings in his chest, sensing the awakening, drawing air into the lungs himself. Sweet flavor of life. Breathing. Without help.

Now it was time to peg in on breathing's sister target: swallowing. After that, there would be other rivers to cross. Less formidable. Slurred speech, drooping eyelids, arm and hand weakness. But the big one had been forded, and he knew for sure he'd cross them all and walk out of that room restored.

Viewed from the perch of the present, it was easier to understand where he had then stood in his pilgrimage. Details of his treatment and progress were easier to discuss. The doctor talked as freely as the patient's ear could tolerate. And this was beneficial therapy. All things pointed to recovery, but a little flag went up on the far hill. The myasthenic drew a deep breath and told himself that more than faith was called for now.

Personal good works can be very important. Let the patient cheat a bit on his self-care instead of calling on the nurse to handle it. Let him try to bathe himself, in spite of wobbly legs and inability to bring arms around body enough to swab shoulders and backside. Lift the left hand with the right when the left is too weak to lift itself. How else can the face be soaped and shaved? Let him comb his own hair (he wasn't half getting bald), even if getting those hard-rubber teeth to the scalp is a major project.

And when the fluids and secretions build up in the chest enough to make breathing difficult, don't let the call bell be the first reaction. Slip on the rubber gloves, clear the catheter from its antiseptic kimono, use the bed-table mirror to locate the trach-tube opening without hit-or-miss fumbling, poke the tube into your own dear chest, and suck the secretions out yourself.

From the hospital's point of view this is definitely a no-no. From the recovering patient's locus, a minivictory. The old morale gets a gutsy boost. The myasthenic knew he was coming along fine when he could handle himself this way. But as with much in this world, there are dangers in taking things into one's own hands.

Somehow it was inward-warming when the duty nurse came into the room and caught him in the act.

"You *know* you're not supposed to be doing that!" adjusting the granny glasses at a severe angle in an unsuccessful attempt to add authority to her words. "*You're* going to get it!"

He pulled the catheter out of his throat, deflated the cuff and plugged the trach-tube with his forefinger.

"You're prettier than a picture when you're mad." The trach-tube made his voice raspy. "That pants suit does something special for you. Model it for me. Come on. Turn around. Slowly now."

Fresh and dewy. Warm and loving. A joy for any eyes, tired or otherwise. Excitingly lumpy where female lumps should be. Victorious over the trim formality of the costume. Geraldine was a doll.

A flush warmed her cheeks at his admiration. She almost stamped her foot as she turned back to him, insisting on her official position.

"All right. All *right!* You *know* you mustn't do it. You'll get infected and I'll have twice as much to do to take care of you."

It was hard for her to suppress a smile.

"Okay," he lied to her. "I'll never do it again."

Both of them knew he would.

The day they took the breathing-machines out of his room for good, another happy incident occurred. His sister and her husband, his first family visitors, came to see him. Until then he'd had to make do with his wife's regular letters and funny get-well cards, since he had insisted that the overnight trips from Connecticut to visit him were too tough for her to take.

George and Louise had driven out from California. It was an intense delight to see them, even though his inhibited speech was a torment. The weak muscles were making his voice slur and fade out. With his visitors facing him in that antiseptic room he wanted nothing more than to be able to talk up a storm. But a few sentences, even a few words at times, would jam the speech machinery and he'd sound worse than a falling-down drunk. What cruel denial. He liked to talk. Liked? He loved it. And this was the first time in his life he had been seriously denied. By now he had learned to do what could be done. With pad and pencil and wild charade gestures he was able to close the gap. The gossip and jokes and chatter tumbled over each other in giddy fashion. The nurses were introduced to his family. Mutual-admiration societies were born. For more than an hour the room was a social whirl. The patient was the center of attraction and he loved every minute of it. The excitement might not have been too medically beneficent, but it sent his morale higher than a kite.

When the visitors finally had to say good-bye and went off on their way west, he fell back in the easy chair, exhausted, and slept for two hours, deeply undisturbed.

CHAPTER 18

TLC.—American colloquialism

WHATEVER else might have happened to the myasthenic while he'd been confined to his bed, he wasn't going to be afflicted with that ulcerated evidence of neglect, bedsores. Not only was he frequently turned from side to side and given soothing back-rubs, but there was that doughnut of heavy, pliant, emulsified fat. It felt like living flesh to the touch. During his first weeks at the Clinical Center they'd hoicked him up and tucked that comfort-able cruller under his arse, giving him ease for hours longer than any other pad he'd rested on. Very costly substance, he'd heard. A couple of hundred dollars for an eighteen-square-inch piece. Seemed like a hefty price tag. But who's to argue? His *derrière* was madly in love with it.

There were other welcome easements. Frequently, without his having to ask, the duty nurse would turn his pillow or, when he'd been sweating, put on a fresh case and change his johnny-coat. When the bed became unusually soggy, as it often did dur-ing the early days on the ward, she'd sponge-bathe him and dress the bed in fresh linen. And it wasn't all that easy to tuck in the folds of sheet and blanket, roll Old Lump Body back and forth so that she could pull out, smooth the coverings, and corner them in. Some of the nurses could make a body-occupied bed that would have delighted a barracks sergeant's heart.

The myasthenic's lips never cracked at the Clinical Center,

as they'd done in other hospitals. Before they could get dry enough to split and his mouth went foul as the bottom of a parrot cage, the nurse would seem to sense the impending discomfort and bring on the soothing, lemon-glycerine swabs.

Not infrequently, going about their room-chores, the nurses would press his hand in passing and smile and maybe say something pleasant. And they'd chatter with him about their own concerns. There was the very young daughter who was living with the boy who wanted to marry her but whom she refused in defiance to "The System." And the entire family joy in the new British bicycles which rode so smoothly through Rock Creek Park on the Sundays. And pleasure at praise for the pretty good writing in the PTA house organ that was edited by one of the nurses in her spare time. No world-shattering confidences. Just people things.

One of the patient's nurses was a tall, enormously healthy girl who enjoyed naughty badinage. It was a little past midnight and her duty tour was over but she'd stayed on to do him a special service.

"You're a dear and I'm much obliged to you," he said. "But I'll bet you only did it to get on my good side. So's I wouldn't give you a hard time tomorrow."

"Give me a hard time any time and you know what I'll give *you*," she leered verbally.

Since she wasn't a woman given to the cutes, in spite of her act, she usually got away with her penchant for sexy references. Providing they didn't have all their clothes off. Though she mock-invited the chase, had he been able to rise like Lazarus, ancient as either of them might be, she'd have fled in blushing retreat.

"So what'll you give me?" he asked, playing straight man.

"*You'll* find out, if you aren't the best patient this ward ever saw."

"You wouldn't dare, you lovely coward. Besides, how can *I* be the best patient?"

"What do you mean?"

"Everybody knows that the best patient is the millionaire with the positive Wasserman. And I ain't even rich."

She threw back her head to let the hearty laugh run free. What she wanted to say didn't come easy to her tongue, so she extended her right hand, as men do when they meet. Her grip was firm. It was a gesture the patient had never seen another woman make in quite that way. Beth did it repeatedly.

The call over the intercom pulled her out of the room. They were busy on the ward that night and she delayed her departure for another hour. When she came back with the night's wrap-up medication, he made mock fuss at not getting his potassium and Maalox on time.

"Like I told you before, I'm not taking any nonsense from you this night," in an avenging-angel voice. "You're doing an awful lot of complaining. What do you expect *me* to do about it?"

"Crawl in here and keep me warm," he suggested.

She extended her hand to him.

"Dreamer."

Nurses are more than women in uniforms. Dust from the fields they work in settles on most of them, like a provocative scent. They come in all sizes, shapes, and dispositions. They evoke a wide range of reactions.

There are plain women, whose teeth and sallow skin are not their happiest features but who literally become physically attractive as they go about their work. And there are few sights of more delight to the masculine eye than wriggly bottoms of nubile nurses sashaying underneath starched skirts. Pants suits on the ward can be as attractive as practical. Most of the women wore them to considerable cosmetic advantage. But to the myasthenic, the prototypical nurse was always costumed in skirt and jaunty cap. The most attractive one he'd ever seen was a nurse who'd attended him on his arrival. There was a serene softness about this young woman's face. Light eyebrows arched angularly. Mouth sensuous and inviting. High forehead framed by ash-blonde hair that cushioned the cap perched squarely atop her head. That starched tiara, held in place less by concealed pins than by the way she carried herself, was a simple white linen circlet, not much bigger at the bottom than a coffee cup, widening an inch or so at the top, four inches high. Not every nurse could have worn such a cap. It was as if she had excited the imagination of a talented designer and he had created it for her.

Her body was a sensualist's dream. Wasp waist. Generous breasts. Full hips. Well-shaped legs, with patrician ankles. Her walk, naturally unhurried, moved her in and out of the sickrooms in a smooth and elegant manner. She was a gentle woman and spoke in a clear and quiet voice that was singularly musical. She exuded sex naturally and not by design. The sick man was saddened by his attraction for her. Too very bad the clock could not be turned back. But even the wildest ego flight could not regard his aged body as other than an insurmountable barrier.

When he had recovered enough to go out onto the grounds to walk with some strength, she had come along with him and had talked about many things. A special interest of hers was airplanes. She was an avid aerophile, sad that her nurse's purse was not fat enough for more flying lessons.

"Two more and I'll solo."

He had the good sense to refrain from any reference to angels.

Try as they will to avoid it, some nurses become emotionally involved with their patients. This subjective relationship can be particularly rough when the nurse must sit for long hours with the terminal sufferer who is floundering around for help before the thread is cut.

All problems involving the nurses ultimately center in the office of the head nurse. At the Clinical Center she was a quiet, easy-moving woman who seemed taller at first meeting than she actually was. Military bearing does that, sometimes. It was her responsibility to deliver silk-smooth nursing service to the two fifth-floor wards, and this she did with the deceptive ease of the professional.

One of her major problems, she had told the myasthenic, was staff morale. On this quiet morning, when she'd brought in his medication herself so she could check him against the charts and her own observations, the subject arose again.

"You look a little on the glum side," he'd remarked, by way of greeting. " 'Smatter?"

"One of those days," she replied, handing him the respirometer to check the liter capacity of his lungs.

Dutifully he sucked in as much air as he could and slowly exhaled it through the small machine to the very last gasp. The tiny arrows spun around their dials to show a fairly creditable 2.5 liters. For his height, 3.6 would have been normal. Still, that 2.5 was a deal better than the showing he had made the week before.

As he handed the device back to her, he said, "It can't be all that bad, surely."

Mary Thompson, professional nurse, U.S. Army Corps colo-

nel, active reserve, with a generous helping of that cement between doctor, nurse, and patient that holds most of medicine together, weighed her response. Her tone was deliberate and a little
sad.

"Shirley Moss is leaving."

Shirley was one of his favorites. She'd been part of the duty
crew that had welcomed him to the Clinical Center.

"Why does she want to leave? Family troubles or something?"

He was sure it would have to be a big deal. She had seemed
to him happy and contented in her job. But the sick man had
seen only one side of a many-faceted pattern. There had been no
apparent crisis, no accident that might have shaken her unduly.
In any case, had there been, she would have handled it ably. She,
like her head nurse and many of her sisters, was not a woman
given to flap.

Shirley had come to work that morning as usual, walked
down the hall to the nurses' station, past the children in their
wheelchairs, their bandaged heads in crash helmets, and looked
around the ward as if she were seeing it for the first time. Im-
munity against sharing the torments of her charges, so painstak-
ingly developed, had vanished in thin air.

Shirley Moss had walked down the hall to the head nurse's
office, said she had to leave, returned to her ward and worked
out the shift as if nothing untoward had happened. Then she
went home. There was a lot of Latin language in the diagnosis,
but it translated to "nervous breakdown."

"It's a serious problem for us in spite of the advantages here,"
the head nurse said, scratching some figures on the myasthenic's
chart. "After all, we're here for research. We get more complicated and serious diseases here to cope with than they do in the
private hospitals. It isn't that we aren't patient-oriented. But having to look after the sick people here gets grim sometimes for
some of the nurses."

It was clear that while cure is the primary aim of the private
hospital, at such research facilities as the Clinical Center, it is
only a side effect. They are geared to learn from one to help
many. That's why their nurses seldom see the cures that make
the work rewarding.

What she'd said about the private sector had recalled his
floor doctor's remark that the happiest people in medicine are
those concerned with bone trauma. Set a bone and you know

what to expect. There are very few surprises of any kind. The bone knits up and the patient gets well again. Even infectious diseases are usually handled without too many problems.

Mary Thompson smiled as she said, "You can see why we're all so happy when we see that somebody we've nursed has recovered and gone home and then come back to visit us."

CHAPTER 19

*Physicians are those upon whom we set our hopes when ill;
our dogs when well.—Ambrose Bierce*

ONE of the nights when the ward was quiet and the doctor didn't
have a date, he came into the myasthenic's room to check on his
patient before going home.

"How are you feeling? Swallowing any better today?"

"About the same, I think. Can't seem to get off this stupid
plateau. Don't tell me there isn't anything you can do about it."

"Well, we've been thinking of trying Mestinon. It might
give the muscles the boost they need."

"Be my guest. When do we start?"

"Soon. We'd like to wait a little longer."

The patient grumbled at the delay. It was like the movie
business in the old days: Hurry up and wait. Same today, of
course. But he reined in plaint. They probably wanted to give
the prednisone a bit more time to do its stuff.

"You've tried Mestinon with the prednisone, haven't you?"

"No. In the other two patients we used prednisone alone.
They improved, so we didn't have to add Mestinon. Glad we
didn't. Use two different drugs and you're never sure which did
what."

"Could Mestinon react badly on me?" the myasthenic
wanted to know.

"Could be. It's a risk."

"Won't be the first one."

"Nor the last."

"How about lab tests? I read somewhere that there's a rabbit with myasthenia. Maybe you could try it on him. You've heard about this Bugs Bunny, haven't you?"

He had. The report had been circulated in Sunday supplements and various journals because of the prevelant belief that there is no satisfactory laboratory animal for the study of myasthenia gravis.

The story was that the bunny's ears drooped in a king-size ptosis but could be restored to their normal erect position through administration of anticholinesterase chemicals. B'rer Rabbit's life-span may have been diminished by the laboratory experiments he had been subjected to. That wasn't very important to anybody but the rabbit. What did matter was that when he had fulfilled his days and gone to that Great Cabbage Patch in the Sky, his thymus gland (common to man and many domestic animals) and neuromuscular functions had been dispatched for inspection by skilled technicians. One of these scientists, if the term in this case is not too distantly employed, doused the bit of bunny with a destructive chemical. To err is human. And that was the end of that.

"There's a dog somewhere that's a myasthenic, too, isn't there?"

"Don't know about the dog," the doctor answered. "But he isn't the only hope. One of the immunologists here, a year or so ago, did some work with guinea pigs. Nonhuman variety." He smiled.

"What happened?" the patient was eager to know.

"His work supported the hypothesis that the myasthenic's body itself inflames the thymus."

"How?"

"Don't know. But if you can extract a certain protein from the thymus and inject it into cavies or rats, you get a neuromuscular block that resembles the myasthenic pattern. But they aren't the ideal animal models, either."

"I was told in New York that man is the only adequate lab animal for MG."

"That's right. He is. Ideal. Though some animals look promising. They've been able to develop polymyositis in animal models."

"Which is?"

"Muscle inflammation. Myocarditis, too. Heart muscle. There's a new technique circulating antibodies to striated muscles found in about a third of all myasthenics."

"Striated?" the man asked.

"The voluntary muscles are striated. Striped. Grooved."

"Groovy."

The doctor upped an eyebrow.

"I think I'm keeping you up too late. That had overtones of a relapse."

"Sorry about that," laughing lightly. Then, serious again, "If you had to come up with an educated guesstimate, how long before myasthenia can be cured? Really cured?"

The doctor studied the question for a long minute.

"No more than ten years. Could be sooner. If the disease is caused by a virus, sooner or later it will be identified. When we find out what it is we'll come up with a preventive. That's the only real cure. A preventive."

"Ten years seems like an awful long time, considering how much is already known."

The doctor settled lower into the big chair.

"Ten years isn't really very long. You have to remember that myasthenia gravis is a unique disease. The only one similar to it is the Eton-Lambert syndrome, where a tumor seems to be responsible for the neuromuscular block. It isn't an easy malady to handle, myasthenia. I like the idea of culturing thymus tissue from myasthenics with a new technique to extract a factor that produces that same kind of block. If we can define the substance that causes the block, we'll be at the cause. Or close to it."

"Speed the day," the myasthenic prayed. "And good luck."

That was enough of that and they began to talk grab-bag, as people do when they get on together and want to push acquaintance a little closer to friendship.

Though these two men were associated in that most intimate relationship shared by doctor and patient, there hadn't been much time to get to know each other. There were other barriers, less vulnerable than the Great Wall of China and not likely to be easily breached. Old men and young men seldom think they have as much in common as they actually do. And, too frequently, men of all ages impatiently run before they manage to walk well. The pool is usually where they expect it to be, so they hare across the lawn and launch themselves—without checking the water level. A man can get easily hurt doing that.

The doctor settled lower on his spine and laced his fingers behind his head. The quiet sigh said it had been a busy day. To the invalid it seemed an ideal opportunity to probe this sophisticated segment of the younger generation on more than medical matters.

"I wish we were in a congenial saloon tonight. Not a noisy one. A talk saloon. Most of the world's problems are solved in saloons."

"This might be a good night for it. I could do with a drink or two about now, too."

"Since I'm room-bound, how's about writing a couple of spiritus frumenti orders?"

"I'd get my head on a plate."

"Pity. I guess we'll have to make do with something less tasty. For openers, how do you stand on the cause and effect issue? Or the vice versa, if you want to dive into the deep end right away."

If they'd been on the weed or were actors playing a scene, this was the time the doctor would have fired up a cigarette, dawdling the lighting of it, to sort of break up the dialogue and make the question appear to have more meat than was actually on its bones.

"I had a professor once who liked to worry things like that," the young man said. "He was an either-or addict. Claimed it was a mistake to see all either-ors as unsatisfactory."

The patient said he couldn't agree more. "There come times when simple dichotomy serves the purpose better than anything else, I think."

The shadow of garrulity began to fall across the room. But there's pleasure in that at times. The sick man was enjoying the company and the talk.

"I think we live in a chancy world," he said. "A head-or-tail proposition. Blind chance peoples the globe. No, it really does," as the doctor smiled. "It gives us two kinds of people. Superior and inferior. Confucius say same thing."

The pause was transient. His smile went as broad as limp muscles would allow.

"I wouldn't hold strong on that superior-inferior doctrine if I weren't absolutely sure *we* fit into guess what category."

He had come to this binary concept a long time ago. When he'd found out that it had been expressed a couple of thousand years ago by the Chinese sage, he'd been pleased he'd thought of it. Not that he'd had any idea this view had been original with him.

"History clearly demonstrates," he argued, "that there are few of mark and many of common run. I suppose we ought to find a more suitable word than 'inferior.' 'Commonplace' is probably just as offensive to the umbrage-takers. But old Ma Nature sure shows her profligacy with people just as she does with salmon eggs."

Nobody knows what sets this one on one side and that one on the other, but the two men agreed that neither wealth nor position separate the goats from the sheep.

"What actually does it is what most people hate like hell to accept. Luck or fortune or lot or hazard. Call it what you like."

It was his adamant belief—everybody is "ismed" one way or another—that it was a mighty coin-flip, an Olympian pot-luck that determined the nature and the raw material quality of every babe that's born. Some make it, whatever the goal. Some don't. Just like salmon eggs. Very few of those laid ever learn to swim.

By this time the philosophical clock was running down. The doctor looked at his watch.

"It's getting late. You'd better get some sleep."

"I think I will," the patient said, all of a sudden tired. "See you tomorrow. And many thanks. For everything."

CHAPTER 20

◆§ *Defend me from busy doctors.—Welsh proverb*

INABILITY to communicate with his fellows is one of man's grimmest burdens. Failure to word-frame thoughts and emotions adequately has pushed the human animal into all manner of nasty practices.

Lying flaked-out in a myasthenic sickroom is a lot less grim than warfare but it can be pretty rough on the invalid who has to try to get through to people with crude gestures, ineffectual shruggings, and idiotic rolling of the eyeballs. This presumes that the patient is on an artificial respirator and can't talk and is too weak to hold a pencil and write.

The problem of this kind of sickroom communication isn't new. During the past several years a variety of mechanical devices have been introduced to cope with it. One such, in use on 5-East ward, had been built by the Fairchild-Heller Company. It was about a yard square and three or four inches deep, standing on end like a Manhattan glass-steel building, marked off into a number of little windows bearing such legends as "Too Cold," "Close Door," "Radio On," "Mouth Swab," and the like. The slightest pressure on the button at the end of a long cord would light up the desired windows.

Cousin to the windowed box was the "Speak-Easy," a circular device that bore the alphabet and numerals around its outer rim; words and phrases around the two inner circles. The three arrows, one for each circle, could be moved forward or backward by the slightest touch on the small control-board buttons. And if the hand muscles were dormant, it could be operated by a head-band through which the brow muscles controlled the pointers.

Cards with key words and phrases, usually tailored to the individual patient's needs, were sometimes Scotch-taped to the bed's guard rails. The patient pointed to whatever was wanted.

But no scheme or device could possibly be an adequate substitute for a real-live, sympathetic nurse who is adept at mind-reading. Such a paragon could make palm-talk almost an adventure. The Connecticut myasthenic learned this very old communications system early in his illness.

In palm-talk the nurse rests her dear hand, palm up, under your index finger. Assuming you know most of the alphabet and can spell a little, you trace in her palm the first letter of the first word of your message. Say it's an "f." Trace "f" on that soft, lightly lined plain. (She's a young nurse.) She says "f." You make an okay sign with your eyes or you head-nod, whichever comes first, and then go on to the next letter: "e." She gets it and says so. You do another "e" but maybe you hurry it. She isn't sure. So you make a wiping erasure motion across her palm and retrace the "e." Now she calls it. You go on to the "t" and make the sign the word is ended. The angel says, "Feet."

A true blow for liberty has been struck.

The nurse, being a bright and imaginative lassie, goes at once into binary questioning. When the patient can't talk, no nurse worth her Epsom salt will ever ask such silly questions as "Do you want a blanket or to have your pillows turned?"

Knowing now that "feet" is on the patient's mind, the nurse asks, "Feet cold?" A yes-nod. "Want a blanket?" A no. "Bed-socks?" The light in the invalid eyes tells her she has cut the knot. And when, with the sweet suggestion of a knowing smile, she adds, "How's about a feet-rub first?"—incarnate paradise.

On such occasions, the myasthenic desperately wanted to give her, as a totally inadequate token of his appreciation and affection, three floor-length minks and open accounts at Bergdorf's and Tiffany's. It is no minor matter to have luxurious massage and wool bed-socks to warm icy feet and let sleep slip over you.

The warm and compassionate nurse, long a sickroom veteran who had brought these special comforts to his bed, one quiet, feet-rub night had noted the overlong toenails and suggested a pedicure. That chiropodic attention was worth a trip to Fort Knox with a shopping bag. And when she and her sisters took time out from the ward chores to give him sybaritic back-rubs, heaven held no greater rewards.

There were other lesser pleasures at this home away from home. Get-well cards, most of them, were welcome. A few of them amused the nurses, but they were a tough audience, having seen so many. The coyly suggestive ones produced more bored disapproval than moral indignation. Letters were more welcome than cards, of course. More can be said. But all mail to the ailing tapers off fairly quickly after the spate at the outset of confinement. Then they dwindle, trickle, and stop altogether. Except for a word now and again from the faithful. Maybe a scheme could be devised, he said one day to the duty nurse, whereby the welcome mail would arrive at regular intervals throughout the entire time the patient has to spend in hospital.

One early afternoon, after feasting on three long and newsy letters, he had leaned back in the large chair and semidozed. It was a tranquil loll. But some camel's nose always seems to poke at the tent flap. A piercing pain struck his hand. A hot needle had been rudely thrust into the base of his palm, where it joins the wrist. He jerked in reflex and rubbed the spot briskly. The pain persisted strong enough to force sweat-beads on the forehead and underarms and to press him to catch up his breath. It seemed much longer (as such things often do) than the seconds it took to ease off and disappear. What had sent that message to that specific spot? Why? And what was the message? If any.

Hadn't the doctors said that pain is not part of myasthenia?

Things happen without purpose. At times it seems so. The all-knowing knows, whoever he (or she or it) is, must be aware that this is a chancy world.

The elders in the myasthenic's family used to say that idle hands are the devil's workshop. This tenet seemed to be highly endorsed at the Clinical Center by the occupational-therapy ladies. It was their job to distract the patients from their maladies. The OT females would come on to the wards with all manner of artful and distracting notions. Paint a seascape by the numbers. Paste sequins into glittering peacocks. Thank the powers no one suggested painting on black velvet, a sin worse than genocide.

There was offered the opportunity to plait a leather belt or hook a rug. He had a belt. So he opted for the rug.

That's how he got acquainted with Judy. She was in occupational therapy. And belonged in occupational therapy like you need a finger in your ear on the Easter Parade. But she was earning her buck and so she sweet-talked him into trying a rug. Rug-hooking is not a mentally taxing exercise, although it does require a certain amount of manual dexterity. That was all to the good. It stirred up the hand and finger muscles.

He and the pretty put their heads together—she smelled delicious—and went through the stock book of rug designs. He didn't think he cared for the tiger. The Early American eagles were designed to ensure their inability to fly. The sleeping spaniels and the floral designs were as exciting as wet Quaker Oats.

"Why don't you do your own?" she suggested. It was a question with only one answer for an egoist. So he did. It came out to be a sunburst in a creamy field bordered by two shades of green. Some might have preferred the tiger.

Whatever the design, rug-hooking is a good deal like eating peanuts. Fun to do. Once started, hard to stop. It not only ate up time but furnished a small esthetic satisfaction. He was glad he had discovered it. Some people take all the credit.

Without warning, one pleasant, balmy afternoon when he was getting on so well, the blow was struck. It was in the hands. They had been strong and flexible for so many days that he'd completely forgotten their earlier failures. Maybe that piercing pain that had stabbed his hand the other day had been the warning. Whatever it was, his hands and fingers had been reduced to sporadic immobility again.

No pain. But no control. He would hook a few strands of wool into the netting and that would be it. He would have to put the hooking tool aside and rest his hands. It took minutes, always more in his mind than a stopwatch would have recorded, before he could pick up a dingly bit of colored yarn, drape it around the hook and pull it into place.

The muscle failure in his hands wasn't even in the ball park with such difficulties as inability to breathe or swallow. But to the sick man it was nearly as savage a blow.

He had been getting on so well. Without actually framing the words, he told himself he had been on the way home. He made a definite point to himself that the wicked, debilitating disease had been tamed by the prednisone's St. George. But it had escaped its cage and was loosed, like the hounds of war, on his body once again. Cutting his hands off at the wrists might well be no more than Act One. That he might be going down again instead of up, that he might be beaten into that vegetable state that was his greatest fear were possibilities keen enough to churn his stomach into a sour brew. The nurse brought in antacid, but he knew well enough that nothing in the entire world outside himself could diminish his shock one bit.

Quietly he pulled himself together. Despite the disappointment of the hand failure, it was not so dramatic as other milestones in his illness had been. It must have been being caught unaware that made the shock so sharp. The sudden defeat of great expectations has the makings of panic in it.

Five full minutes went by before he moved his hands again to pull snippets of yarn into the rug. Hands and fingers responded normally. But he was not deceived. Three or four hookings, maybe half a dozen, and the muscles again refused. Another waiting. Five minutes more. Five long minutes before he could again outrassle a little piece of colored yarn. That's a long time. Try holding your breath. Count it out. You'll never make five minutes. It is a hell of a long time. And frustration stretches it a lot further than that.

There were other flies in the ointment about this time, too. Recurrences of diplopia and ptosis. He didn't like the ptosis, but it was copable. It was the double vision, bringing on blurry weakness and excessive watering to the eyes, that denied much of the wonderful world of the printed page. Garden-variety diplopia wasn't the worst thing in the world. He could always hold a hand over one eye. But blurry eyes don't read well.

Strengthened by his battle with the faltering fingers, he sat out the eye bout without too much fuss. As with all things, that too passed away. Four days later. And in its passing he could have his books again. Praise be to all the gods for that, from Allah through Cronus to Zeus, with Nut thrown in for piquancy.

By proxy he had combed the shelves of the patients' library, which later he was to visit with great pleasure, and so he never wanted for good books. When the urge for "constructive" reading nibbled at him, he brushed up on his French, dived into biographies, or turned to reference works to pry further into the subtleties of his disease.

Delighting in the way words can roll around on the tongue and caress the ear, it was easy to become beguiled by medical argot. Could be, he was inclined to think, that the strongest wall around doctors, lawyers, and priests is their cant. The little old proverb-maker was probably right when he observed that in the presence of the patient the language is always Latin.

The myasthenic wasn't all that long into his malady before he'd had a nodding acquaintance with such words as "dysphagia," which almost sounds like swallowing disability; "diplopia," which is much gussier than double vision; and "dysphonia," a pleasant sound describing talk trouble. Words like these have a certain acoustic charm and perhaps a pinch of mystery, but they aren't easy to work into the average dinner conversation.

At some cocktail party in the future, he fancied himself making a wave or two by remarking that the latest bestseller seemed to him to be "marasmic," which is a second cousin on its mother's side to "flaccid," "flabby," and "feeble." Maybe with one more than his alcoholic quota under the belt, he might even try "pneumomediastinography."

"Fasciculation," as any etymologically precocious child well knows, refers to the twitching of a group of fibers. It doesn't come up often but in certain circles it could almost be used as a dirty word.

Picking his way gingerly through this vocable minefield, he made note of words that could never be used without a stethoscope *in situ* and scalpel in hand, but which had charming and delicious sounds. Try "parethesia," "myalgia," or "ophthalmoplegic myasthenia" at the next barbecue burn-in. They'll get more respect than's deserved.

In the neuro section of one of the medical books, he was fascinated to learn that the sixth cranial nerve turns the eyes to the outside. Good thing for drill sergeants to know, he mused. The third cranial nerve turns the eyes inward and, for a bonus, contracts the pupils. Number seven—lucky or unlucky, however it happens to the dicer—makes laughter and weeping possible. And without the fifth cranial, William Wrigley would never have had enough money to buy a Pacific Ocean island off the shores of Southern California. The fifth triggers chewing. The twelfth controls the tongue. But not often enough. It is the villain which, when failing, plays hob with speech. The ninth and tenth handle swallowing, unless myasthenia has taken hold, and then they don't handle swallowing.

Maybe all this was quite true. Maybe it wasn't. But the book said it was, and there is a tremendous power in the printed word. The printed word becomes the father of undeniable verity as a result of a little ink filmed over a bit of metal and pressed onto a piece of paper. In a hardcover book the word becomes gospel.

The myasthenic, in these medical explorations, never did get into skeletal country. Anklebone connected to the legbone. Legbone connected to the thighbone. Maybe it was just as well. A very long time ago, anatomy had been one of his electives at Loyola College. He couldn't remember why. At any rate there didn't seem to be time enough left over from basketball, the bass fiddle, and girls for the course to make much of an impression. About all he could remember was that the greater trochanter of the femur articulates in the acetabular cavity of the ischium. Or is it the os inomynatum?

Reading the dictionary was always rewarding. It washed out a lot of sitting-there time that he might have otherwise found difficult to fill. Words are deceptive instruments. No doubt about that. Misused and abused so much more often than not. Mainly so, he thought, when venality is not the spur, because the accepted forms of speech and grammar are not mastered before they are waved aside for invalid substitutes.

He remembered his Jesuit mentor trying to impress upon him the importance of mastering a discipline before being entitled to outrage it. Invent and neologize as you will, but not until you know what changes you are ringing on the bells. There are laws. No matter who is head of state, who the prettiest girl in town, what bank holds the mortgage on the farm—a sonnet is intransigent. It must have fourteen lines. No more. No less. Or it ain't a sonnet.

Hours passed pleasantly with these cerebral gambols, during which he didn't once think about himself or his problems. Which didn't hurt the healing process. So, if one is indisposed and words aren't one's cup of tea, it would be wise to try something else for diversion. Anything to take one outside oneself.

The occupational-therapy ladies might be right, at that.

CHAPTER 21

I owe much. I have nothing.
I give the rest to the poor. —Rabelais

THERE comes a time when it is sensible to think about the disposition of one's worldly goods. Each of us has something to be left behind, even if it is only a cadaver.

The Connecticut myasthenic's will had been written long enough ago to warrant updating. Both his wife and his sister knew his views on funerals and memorial services, of which he wanted neither. The services he had attended, for a variety of reasons but only one of them for pleasure, didn't seem to him to be the most desirable way to bid the dear departed bon voyage. After all, he was already gone.

Usually, on the days of these services, there was an assembly in front of some chapel, small-talking until the doors were opened, as if it were coming up curtain time. Once inside, there would be some organ music of indistinct character, and a man would come onstage, adjust the lectern, face the congregation, and clear his throat. There would be language about giveth and taketh away, and laudatory remarks about a person he may never have met in life. On signal the people would stand or kneel or sit, most of them not knowing what it was for. After a while the minister or pastor or rabbi or priest or reader would snuff out the candles. People would file out. On the sidewalk something would be said about the deceased and plans would be made for the rest of the day. And that would be that.

He realized his views were narrow, picky, and selfish. He reckoned he was mildly entitled, since he had never even nudged anybody to go along with him. It was just that he didn't want anything like that for himself. Better to get his body to the nearest medical school (for which he had made provision in the will) where, he hoped, a student or two might learn, outside the bedroom, something about the way the human anatomy is chunked together.

Eyes and kidneys and other usable viscera, unless the myasthenia canceled that out, might go to people in need of the organs. And maybe, when the practical matters had been tended to, a clutch of his club members might gather at the bar, put down a few drinks, and say something pleasant about him. He might also be remembered for a little while by those relatives and friends he had not too severely outraged. Immortality, he was convinced, is no more than somebody's memory.

Off and on, ever since he had been in the ICU ward at Mt. Sinai Hospital, in April of 1970, his hearing had been giving him trouble. For some reason he was never able to determine, liquids had built up in his inner ears through the action of the mechanical respirator he had been hooked into at the time. He wasn't sure of the name. Cunningham, maybe. After he'd been on the machine for a few days the pressure had been strong enough to block hearing and produce considerable discomfort. After a while it turned to pain. Acute. And constant.

He would not soon forget the morning they called in the ear specialist, who banged the tuning fork for him and looked into his head through a little inverted funnel. After the examination he was told the eardrums would have to be pierced to release the liquids. His stomach jumped a foot. Stick a needle into his eardrums? The very thought of it was excruciating. But he got a break. He never had to find out how much that kind of thing can hurt. Before they got around to the piercing he was transferred down to General Care, where he went onto the Bird respirator. Mysteriously, the pressure eased in his ears and needles were never used. But the ringing remained. Tinnitus is the doctor-word for that constant quiet roaring, as when a conch is held to the ear.

At the Clinical Center, when he became ambulatory, he wondered if maybe something could be done about that humming. They sent him down to the ear clinic. Sound-and-speech tests were made. There was a definite hearing loss at two thousand cycles, a lack of sound distinction and discrimination—fine tuning, they called it—at those levels. The trouble could be caused by advancing age, heredity, and degeneration of the acoustic nerves. Add to that the possibility that some of his medication tended to restrict the otic arteries. Part of the tinnitus might have been caused by the sound of blood rushing through constricted blood vessels.

In sum, the test doctor told him that his hearing problem was progressive, that hearing aids wouldn't do any good, and that he might as well settle down and live with it. He settled. For a while. It was in New York, months later, when he was with people again and could get around under his own steam, that he'd gone to a highly recommended ear specialist for another opinion. Silly bastard. Not the ear man. Him. Would have done better to believe the NIH people. But he was feeling so well generally at that time that he didn't think he was ready yet to say, "Eh? What's that?" to everything.

That visit to the ear specialist had cost him the better part of a hundred dollars. He re-found out that he was getting old in the ears and he'd have to put up with it. The visit did remind him of the old wheeze about the guy who went to the ear doctor with a hearing complaint. The medic examined the man thoroughly and asked the usual questions about liquor and sex.

"Well," says the complainant, "I have a couple martinis at lunch, a few highballs before dinner, maybe a bottle of wine with the meal now and then. Nothin' too much."

"Sex?" the doctor pried.

"I'm married, y'know. We get along okay. Maybe a coupla times a week. Then I got this girl over in Tenafly for the weekends. An' once in a while I run into some of that off-the-path stuff. An' oh yeah. The new secretary—"

The medic did jottings on his prescription pad, weighed and calculated, paused dramatically before delivering the verdict.

"There's no question about it," he said. "You've got to give up all that."

The patient thought seriously about that for a fast minute, stared at the doctor and replied.

"Give it up? Come on, doc. Not just to hear a little better."

CHAPTER 22

❧ *A man in good health is always full
of advice for the sick.—Meander*

THINGS began looking up in April.

The swallowing muscles were still dormant, but there were compensations. Strength was moving back into arms and legs. The doctors, well aware of what happens to muscles that just lie there, had marked his chart for physical therapy. (They seemed to cover all the bases at the Clinical Center.) So, for more than two weeks, a seemingly fragile, sinewy 110-pounder visited him, stretching and twisting his limbs, widening the arc each day to the point of pain twinge, then easing off, only to pull back again until he yipped.

After a few days the dormant muscles responded with a tingling glow of appreciation. It didn't half make him feel good. And the day before the little strong woman said, "Good-bye and good luck," he was able to totter into the bathroom and bathe himself for the first time in months. How sweet it was to climb into the tub, holding onto the safety rails for dear life, and give himself a sensual lick and a promise. His arms weren't strong or limber enough to cover all of the territory, and he had to settle for a damp *derrière*. The nurse, standing by, dried his back and the southern exposure. In another week he could handle the entire bathing exercise all by himself. "Thanks all the same, nurse. I can manage."

He was sitting up and moving about his room most of the

time now. Control was flowing back into hands and fingers. He could write letters again and make decipherable diary notes. And along about the end of the third week one of the nurses took him for a short walk in the grounds, where pink and white dogwoods caressed his eyes and the sweet nature smell of spring greenery was heady perfume.

No question about it now. He was definitely gaining. Stamina was materially increasing. Even the swallowing symptoms had improved enough by the twenty-fourth to allow him to down a glass of orange juice without the world coming to an end. Two days later, following the afternoon walk, he took some milk, a bit of consommé, fruit juice, and a couple of dollops of ice cream, made a happy note in his diary, and went to sleep that night a very happy man.

Then the sun went behind the clouds.

On the fifth of May, for no reason at all except the instability of the disease, he lost almost all swallowing sensations and couldn't get anything down without most or all of it bringing on a hacking, gobbing storm.

Severe headaches, migrainish, came back again. He felt generally miserable when, on the tenth, they sent him downstairs to begin radiation treatment for skin cancer. The squamous cells on his forehead had been widening and the dermatologist thought it was time to do something about it. These rebel cells, he told the myasthenic, originate in the epithelial tissue and are called keratoacanthoma, a frightening name for little scales that look like permanent dandruff.

There was more skin cancer on chest and shoulders, but these outcroppings weren't too serious in the specialist's eyes. The forehead was the main arena.

Supine on the X-ray table, staring up at the huge, ominous roentgen eye above him, he propped up his head on a pillow so that the secretions would drain down his throat while the X-rays were hitting him. The doctor and his assistant fitted the lead shield, cut to expose the cancer patch, cautioned him to remain motionless, left the room, and closed the door. A click came from the control room, a buzz, and for four and a half minutes he took one hundred roentgens. He'd be given a dozen more such treatments before the carcinomic cells were destroyed.

When he went back upstairs the day nurse asked him how it had gone. He tried to tell her, but after seven words his voice slurred into gibberish. He wondered if the X-rays had anything to do with it. More than likely not. Just another unpredictable falloff. So he gave the nurse one of those half-assed brave smiles and made a thumb and forefinger circle that usually means okay.

The next morning the doctors decided to try the risky blast treatment Dr. Peter Ré and he had talked about. They were ready now to see if Mestinon could shove him off the plateau. After several tests, some atropine and twelve milligrams of the cholinergic drug went down the tube into his stomach. By five-thirty his speech had materially improved. Overall strength was sharply improved. He was so excited by this dramatic boost that he couldn't get to sleep until long after the Late Late Late.

Joy did not run unconfined throughout the land for long. The very next day he faded. Back onto the old plateau. They ran the experiment for fifteen days, gradually increasing the drug dose from twelve to sixty milligrams.

It didn't do a bit of good. *Au contraire.* Dysphagia increased, diplopia recurred, circumoral muscles flabbed, pulling his face into a snarl. Swallowing went completely out the window. At such times, frustration is hard to beat down.

The following week it was more of the same, except that cramps and diarrhea had been added. Speech was almost normal, but he didn't have much to say that wouldn't be complaint. And to the larger problems little irritations intruded. Like when, in the bathroom, leaning over to pick up something he'd dropped, his eyeglasses jumped out of his pajama pocket and swan-dived into the toilet bowl. Damn it to hell. Then, less than a hour later, a jigger of gooey antacid slipped somewhere between the nurse's hand and his, cascading all over the book in his lap. Such puky little things can be up-the-wall-sending.

One of them did take on a little drama, though. One night in the middle of July he must have turned the wrong way in bed, scraped the radiation treatment scab off his forehead, and bled like a stuck pig. The crimson flow brought about a basin of nurse attention, which was always welcome. The scab-scrape hadn't hurt a bit and the wound closed over again in a day or so. As he looked at it in the mirror over the washbasin, the new scab had a dry and transient appearance. He simply couldn't resist picking at the incrustation. Instantly, all the way from Connecticut, he could hear his wife's voice, loud and clear.

"It'll never get well if you pick it!"

But he was a man of Jello character. The scab came off easily. In a few more days there was a white island in a wan tan sea. He wasn't too cosmetically concerned, although all of us are sprinkled with vanity dust.

Before the month was out the major battle of the long war was joined inside him. Prednisone against the Invaders.

What tipped the balance will never be known. The body's natural defenses must have rallied, allowing the drug to exert its strongest force. Additional troops from the colonies—the arms and legs, and as far away as the feet—were called up and flung into the fray. It must have been quite a fight. It would have been something to see. After all, it was his body that was the battleground.

Prednisone, plus all his care and therapy, won the day, though it wasn't the kind of conflict where decision came quickly and the enemy fled the field in rout. There was, instead, a certainty of feeling inside him that it was now going to be uphill, a steady drive that would never again be seriously stemmed.

Now the doctors began talking about maybe a change of scenery would do him a power of good. Let him go home for a week or so, nasogastric tube in place notwithstanding. They must have seen the stir-crazy signs before he himself was aware of them. No question but that he was very tired of coop-up. Five months in one room, and most of it in bed, can be wearing.

Since, like old Peg-Leg in the haunting "September Song," he was playing a waiting game—waiting for time and prednisone to put him right—he figured he might just as well play it at Old Greenwich as in Bethesda. It was a happy prospect. Going home would wash away hospitalitis, that chronic, demoralizing drag that builds up in direct ratio to the amount of time under wraps.

Next morning he walked in the grounds for a good half hour. He was closer to the clouds than the greensward, yet halfway around Memorial Road he was jerked back to earth. The pain in his chest came out of left field. He was sure that his breathing muscles, for the first time since he had gone off the respirator, were beginning to weaken. It scared hell out of him. He found a bench and sat very quietly for a long time, almost without moving. The pain went away. Breathing smoothed out. He knew what had done it. He'd walked too rapidly, pressed too hard too soon. Let's take it easy, chum.

Back on the ward, he didn't tell a soul about it. Didn't want to miss going home. August 10 wasn't all that far away.

CHAPTER 23

Illness tells us what we are.—Italian proverb

HE was awake early on that tenth of August.

His wife arrived and helped him cram his clothes, medication, magazines, and diary notes into the travel bag. They brought up a carry-cart for all his gear—the bag, the two-thirds-completed hooked rug, the lush gardenia that had been blooming madly from the very day Doris and his daughter had sent it down to him, months ago.

There were loving good-byes and take-care-y'selfs. He went down the corridor with fairly firm steps, into the elevator, out of the building, and into the Pontiac parked at the curb, exactly one hundred and fifty-seven days after the ambulance had delivered him to this haven.

It was a brisk, bright day for the drive to Connecticut. They took it easy, savored the countryside, stopped just north of Baltimore for lunch. She had people-food—a chicken sandwich. He took his midday medication, filled a gavage bag with formula, hooked it into the NG tube, and let the meal drift into his stomach. Flow gently, sweet Afton.

They were in Old Greenwich by five. No problems. Up the driveway, into the garage. No unloading for him. She wouldn't let him carry anything. And was firm about it. So he went into the house and climbed the stairs to his room. Legs were a bit shaky but solid enough. The cats were glad to see him, judging from the ankle-polishing and harum-scarum scamperings. It was sure good to be home again.

By the twentieth his speech had smoothed out and he was swallowing liquids without aspiration. His wife—always so careful of his diet—cut back on the formula ingredients to maintain the prescribed two thousand calories a day.

Never mind that his tastebuds spurted like artesian wells as he dream-tasted triple-zero Bélons, sluiced down with well-chilled Muscadet; savored heavenly *quenelles de bouchées à la reine;* laid tongue to a rich *bœuf sauté* and any Château-Latour, never mind the year. Then, the flaky luxury of *milles feuilles,* his wife's magnificent coffee, and a fine Napoleon.

Alas, it was a menu that would have to wait. And for more than fattening reasons. Intake had to be carefully watched. Forbidden were cold cuts, fish in oil, rich spaghetti sauces, fried foods. Waffles, sweet rolls, and biscuits were off limits. So were peanut butter, gravies, avocados. Frozen, canned, and preserved fruits were taboo. As for salt—not a speck more than three grams a day. That damned all cheese, except cottage. Cheese is high in sodium and so are all shellfish, except oysters. He was sorry about the cheese but glad about the oysters. Whitstables, Colchesters, Bélons, Chincoteagues, Olympias—what tastebud symphonies.

Happily, wine and spirits were not completely ruled out. Just keep that 2,000 calories in mind. There are 100 in every ounce of whiskey and kindred spirits, half that in an ounce of wine, and 125 in a bottle of beer. All of which would have made his diet rugged to live with, even with his superhuman, indomitable will power. Lucky for him he didn't have to test it. His wife wasn't having any dietary nonsense, so he followed the rules. And liked it.

Just before September showed up he rose early, shaved, showered, and dressed, caught the rattling 10:34 into New York, had his teeth cleaned and checked on Forty-second Street and taxied down Park Avenue to The Players to say hello. It was an enjoyable afternoon. After he'd given himself lunch via the nasal tube in one of the upstairs rooms, he went down and sat for a while in the bar and grill, gossiped some, played a rubber of bridge (badly), and then went up to Grand Central to catch one of the afternoon commuters to Old Greenwich. He was collected by chauffeuse-wife, had a drink and a good dinner. Tired him out, all that activity, but it *was* a happy day.

So was September 10. Breakfast and lunch went well and he knew now that he had it licked. After dinner, where he chewed on a bit of beefsteak, ate the savory veg, and had a glass of Brouilly, he went up to his room and, almost ceremoniously, pulled out the long-irritating nasogastric tube and threw it away. A big and joyful step had been taken.

On September 17 he had been exactly six months on prednisone. He was now taking 175 milligrams every other day, alternating with 30 milligrams. Speech was almost fully normal. Strength and stamina were much improved.

On the twenty-eighth he gave himself a birthday present. He took the tracheostomy-tube out of his throat, plugged the hole with the glass obdurator they'd made for him at NIH for this very occasion, heaved a sigh of relief, and grinned. This, added to the cards and presents and a specially tasty dinner, made it one of the happiest anniversaries he'd ever had.

CHAPTER 24

Visits always give pleasure—if not in the coming, then the going. —From the Portuguese

By November the world was rosy enough to let him go to California. The doctors agreed it would do no harm if he took it easy and was constant with his medication. And the diet. So, ambu bag in hand, he climbed into a 747 and was set down a few hours and a dull movie later at Los Angeles International Airport. It was November 10, 1971.

Who says autumn is a time for decay and dying? It is a time for rhymsters and rhapsodists, a glowing way station in the golden cycle that girdles the sun. California autumn is a very living season. Especially this one.

His sister had his room ready, overlooking the peach tree in the patio. He was greeted deliriously by the poodle, no less warmly but not so unrestrainedly by his sister and her husband. The reunion got off to a good start. He was no longer the scrawny, world-slurring scarecrow they'd seen some months before in Bethesda.

As he moved about the old familiar places there were few corners of that people-packed saucer, tilting off the mountains into the sea, that he didn't know intimately. He'd recognize weathered and weary landmarks and note where the ghosts of others were all that was left. There was a flood of glass and metal buildings, freeways, people, and cars. It wasn't the same old Southern California.

He was diligent with his medication and self-care. A bit looser with the diet. And he did press himself. There were too many and too much to see and be with. Try as he would, overexcitement and underrest usually won the day. The visit was, in a sense, a synthetic three weeks. Trach-care twice a day, medicines at four prescribed hours, lie-downs and chair-rest as often as he would heed his own good sense or his sister's exhortations.

There were a few bad nights and periods of fluctuating strength when the symptoms would return strong enough to give him pause but not enough to make him anxious. He managed. Drugs and determination make a successful formula. Yet, toward the end of his holiday, which, as they always do, came too soon, he was weakening. It was time to go home.

He'd been away from his NIH checkup for some time now. He felt he'd like assurance that the dangers of his disease were miles away and that if they showed their heads, they could be dispelled without too much carrying on. With steroids it pays to keep a watchful eye. Their side effects are not welcome visitors. Cataracts are a serious possibility. And the trained eye can spot the puffiness of face that follows heavy steroid intake. The infallible sign is the buffalo hump that pouches out the soft tissues at the back of the neck between the shoulders.

As his steroid dosage was decreased from the very high levels, five milligrams every three weeks or so, one day the puffiness would go away and excess weight would fall off. High blood pressure levels had to be watched. Normal ranges between 80 and 120. His had gone no higher than 160, which wasn't bad at all. He'd been lucky. Probably was up more than it should have been right then.

So he said his farewells, looked sadly at the hills that were now wearing a thin, gray shroud, mourned the old days, was glad to be going home. The 747 took forty-five seconds to get airborne. They climbed out of the smog-filled basin, banked sharply over the placid sea, pulled up into clean air, and headed east. The day was wet and chilling when they arrived at Kennedy. There were patience-wrecking delays at the ramp and the baggage-wheel. A dull, car-clogged bus ride into Manhattan was followed with the hard-to-take discomforts of the Penn Central that seemed to come with every commuter ticket. He was getting wispy by the time the train staggered into the Old Greenwich station. His wife took him home to a warm house and a three-cat welcoming committee.

As of old, he had overdone it again. Took nearly two weeks to wash out the fatigue. But it had been a wonderful trip.

CHAPTER 25

*The true investigator should have
a robust faith—yet not believe.—Claude Bernard*

THE December 6 visit to Bethesda was a breeze, as such things go. This time he had fancied the train. More reading and lolling time than the airplane. And not all that much longer, door to door.

After the usual taxi hassle at Washington's Union Station, he checked into the Clinical Center and went upstairs. No sooner out of the elevator than the welcoming began. Warm, honey-lamb, old family greetings from "his" nurses, now glad to see him hale and fit. He recalled what the head nurse had said eight months or so before: "The nurses seldom see the victories that make their work meaningful. That's why they're always so glad to see one of their patients who has recovered." That wasn't exactly what she'd said, but it was like enough to make no odds.

The prodigal read into the warmth of the welcome a good deal more than just that. After all, was it not evident to one and all that he was a gay and charming blade in his own right? Autumnal, perhaps, yet withal a measure of dash and élan. The stuff that adventure heroes are made of. Are you listening, Dashiell Hammett? Surely *you* dig it, Ernest H.

So he squeezed and bussed his favorites, helloed from door to door down the corridor, and wound up in his room, where the nurse handed him a gobbet of what couldn't be anything but wallpaper paste, laced with dragon's milk.

"Bottoms up," she said, ever the comedienne.

Two hours later they sent in Mr. Jones, that self-effacing genius with the needle, who could thrust the tiny steel pipe into slippery veins without laying agony on the stickee. They were always drawing blood. Count Dracula should have been so greedy.

A few more tests and the verdict was in. Reduction of the steroid level. Salt-free, low-carbohydrate, two-thousand-calorie diet to continue. Blood sugar level came down. So did blood pressure. The lab report said that his blood was in good shape. Well enough. Inclination to diabetes, which is not unusual in patients who are taking large doses of steroids, makes for slow healing and susceptibility to infection.

Next day they checked for thyroid malfunction. Seems that myasthenics have a higher incidence of thyroid disease than the general public. Thyroid-function blood studies and radioisotope scans usually spot tumors and gland enlargements. Why myasthenics should be abnormally prone to this problem is another one of the not-yet-knowns.

There must be something in MG that reacts with more than normal intensity. It was sharply marked in one of his neighbors on the ward. An attractive girl. Warm, sensitive, very conscious of her appearance, subject to anxieties. Face-muscle limpness and slurred, nasal speech became heavily exaggerated whenever unsettlements were on her. This put oil on the fire. It was a vicious cycle. Sometimes took her a week to recover lost ground.

When his thyroid tests turned out okay it was cancer's turn. It seemed to him a sensible notion to check the over-forties periodically for cancer. His chest X-rays showed a small amount of scar tissue on the left lung, probably from the thymectomy. Otherwise, rodger-dodger.

The test routines were not without their lighter moments. When the myasthenic had bared his manly chest to the EKG technician, the profusion of hair made it difficult for the suction cups to stay in place. One of the operators, who was renowned for her low patience threshold that was just short of magnificent to behold in action, let the first two cups ploop out of place without comment. But when the third let go its hold, she ground her teeth, muttered salty imprecations, and blobbed twice as much goop onto his chest as was necessary to hold the terminals.

She restarted the test by punching the buttons as if the machine was the cause of it all.

"Sorry there's so much hair," he told her. "But since it bugs you when the terminals fall off, why don't you give it up and get into something you might like better?"

She looked at him as if he were daft.

"Give up this job? You crazy, man? I loves it."

A chuckle is a chuckle, wherever it can be picked up.

There were other fish in the pan that demanded attention. He was having a weight problem. He'd gone up to 77 kilograms, which translates to about 170 pounds. It was high enough. Higher than it ought to be, in the doctors' view. Meant having to give up a glass or two of wine and some of the high-calorie dishes that sent his tastebuds into a Southern-belle swoon. But that's life, dearie, he told himself. When it rains over here it shines over there.

The very next day after the poundage conclave, he felt acute neurologic pain stabs on wide areas of his skin. He told himself, with a poor attempt at jocularity, that it was reaction to the talk about his having to give up delicious food and drink. What it actually was was Herpes Zoster, an acute inflammatory disorder of the central and posterior nerve root ganglia. Most of us call it "the shingles." Caused by chicken pox virus, they think—viruses being one of a group of infectious agents. There are three kinds: bacterial, animal, plant. He couldn't tell them apart, even though apparently he had been nipped by the animal-biting variety. After ten days of itching and scratching, and not much laughing about it, Herpes Zoster shoved off.

Finally, there was another session with Big Bertha, the EMG machine that checked his muscle capacity by shocking hell out of it. Those tingling electrical agitations, painful when they came in series, were hardly unbearable. The myasthenic's enormous courage saw him through. Stout lad.

The entire Clinical Center session couldn't have been more agreeable.

Eight days before Christmas they sent him upstairs for just-to-be-sure X-rays. Dutifully he downed not quite an imperial gallon of a revolting barium syrup, bared his hairy chest to the cold eye of the camera, obeyed the "Take a deep breath—hold it!" and snorted like a grampus when he heard the familiar click as the portrait was taken. The short wait for development. Then, good news. There was no serious scarring in the throat from either the thymus operation or the tracheostomy. His swallowing mechanism was in good shape.

From now on, it was up to prednisone and Father Time.

Before it was time to take off for home, he'd gone into Washington and strolled the Mall, visited the Corcoran and lunched with friends, and stopped in at a favorite Japanese restaurant. It was all a breezy holiday.

On top of the favorable test reports were the lashings of euphoria and the sunshine of staff pleasure at his progress. But above it all, he was able to take great relish in the sweet security that comes only when the play is a hit and is likely to run longer than *Life With Father*.

When the EAL jet lifted off the National Airport runway and swung across the Potomac into the leaden sky, the myasthenic felt singularly at peace. No clouds could deny the brightly shining sun. The air was sweeter to the skin, even inside that quivering, noisy tube. And the travel irritants, *in toto*, were sneeze and forget it. He was a lucky man. Alive again. Walking and talking and traveling on his own again. And breathing on his own again, too. NIH had done all this for him. He was much obliged.

What price this pearl?

There was not a trace of ledger blood. None of that crimson ink that withers the resources of the ailing and adds economic catastrophe to major illness. All of the expert care and attention, the scientific skills, the doctorial talent, the manifold services, the entertainments, and divertissements—all of it. As free as the natural beauty of the Clinical Center's grounds. Even laundry and dry cleaning.

For such as this, taxes are never too high.

The holidays that year were singularly pleasurable. It would be hard to top the special Christmas feast his wife prepared. Duck and apple sauce. And brandy-scorched plum pudding. The cats were sure the decorated tree had been hung with gay, colored-glass punching bags just for their own dear delight. Soft music from the Fisher multiplex and the Jansen speakers. The open fire. Peace on this piece of the earth.

The New Year was ushered in again at The Players. Friendly and festive. Corks popped at the appropriate time. One could almost hear a resolution or two being born.

The holidays that year were very gay.

The no-longer-sick man didn't mind going back to Bethesda on January two. Took the shuttle from La Guardia. No problems. Almost like a long commute by this time. The doctors wanted to do some testing before cutting down on the steroid intake again. It was getting to be routine procedure.

He was getting some publicity, too. Just prior to its publication in the *New England Journal of Medicine*, the myasthenic was given an advance copy of the report that Dr. W. King Engels and his deputy, Dr. John R. Warmolts, had written on their prednisone therapy. Some of it was jargon to the lay eye: "Lessening decrement in amplitude of abductor quinti response to twin ulnar nerve shocks 300 m-sec apart revealed that improved neuromuscular synaptic efficiency reached its peak around 12 hours, then ebbed to an overall high level until further improvement followed the next prednisone dose."

Translation: He had done real good.

It also meant he was doing well enough to complain about their reluctance to close the stoma. He figured he'd had that hole in the throat long enough. Their foot-dragging wasn't entirely whimsical. They didn't believe he'd have any more aspiration problems to cope with, but just in case that improbability became fact, it would be easier to deal with it if there was a hole below the Adam's apple into which they could introduce suctioning catheters.

When swallowing is inhibited, food collects in two petal-shaped depressions that lie at the junction of the larynx and the trachea. Normally, the muscles empty these pockets and send the foodstuff on its way. With the muscles dormant, bits of food can get into the windpipe and kick up a storm. Through the hole in the throat they can get at it quickly and snake it out.

His doctors were disinclined to avoidable risk, especially since their star exhibit (at least *he* thought he was) had climbed the ladder so far so well. So he let them talk him out of it again and when he went home, after ten days at the Clinical Center, the glass obdurator was still plugging the stoma.

On April 23 he used the shuttle again to check into NIH for another round of look-see. His report card came up with straight A's, so there didn't seem to be any reason to hold off any longer. May 2 was happy hemstitch day. They gave him a shot of scopolamine, to dry up excess secretions. Apparently he didn't have any secrets they needed truth serum to reveal. They needled some innovar into his arm, preamble to the anesthetic to be administered in the operating room. They wheeled him upstairs and sewed up the hole.

He came home on May 7 and a couple of days later stopped by Greenwich Hospital to show off to the ICU nurses. Dr. Camp snipped out the stitches. A week later you'd have been hard put to see the thin scar-line even if you'd been looking for it.

The beautiful part was that swallowing was as near normal as made no odds. He had been told on several occasions by the experts that the best that can be expected from drugs is 90 percent of normal. Good enough. He was happy to be in the neighborhood.

There was a short fiddle with the prednisone dose in June. He flew down on the twenty-ninth and came home the next day. On the anniversary of his August, 1970, discharge from NIH he was beginning to behave pretty much like a human being again. A couple of times, on clement days, he walked the forty blocks from home to club, strolling comfortably, looking into shopwindows, watching people scurry and scramble in the constant battle with Manhattan's metabolism.

He went to work almost every day. Bought a sport coat on sale at Abercrombie & Fitch. Caught up with the current theatrical books in the Walter Hampden Memorial Library at The Players. Best of these pleasurable pursuits was moving among people again. And being one of them.

Every other day he was taking two fifty-milligram tablets of prednisone, fifty milligrams of potassium chloride, and antacid daily. Not a very high price to pay for his remarkable recovery, though there were a couple of gnats in the amber. His skin was breaking out, mostly around the nose, and he was coming up with the red-eye. Steroids can cause capillary fragility. Several of the tiny blood vessels had ruptured in his right eye. The steroids also increase the output of the sebaceous glands. Oil clogs the pores. Pustules result. A sty came with the package. Could these facial skin problems signal a breaking out of a second youth? Probably not. Alas. Alack.

By the end of September, 1972, he would have completed three months of the hundred-milligram, single-dose, alternate-day prednisone program, and would be coming down five milligrams every three to four weeks, carefully checking reactions.

One fine day in 1973 or 1974 there would be no more prednisone, no more potassium chloride or effervescent tablets, no more antacid. Maybe he'd continue with the multiple vitamin pills. All kinds of healthy people are big on vitamins. Some doctors see them as placebos. Some don't. Not everybody backs the same horse.

But come that day without drugs, when he would be more keenly attuned to living than most of his fellows, it would be difficult to convince this man that at long last they had not found a cure for his incurable disease.

Cure for myasthenia gravis?

Remission?

Containment?

What matter a damn-all how the miracle is named. Who could be sure his disease was not still inside him, banked? Who could be sure it wasn't?

There will come answers to these questions. Responsible answers. In a thousand cubicles across the land men and women are pounding their brains, testing their intuition, taking terminal chances, trying. Trying over and over and over, in the search for solutions. And to aid in the quest there will always be a flow of volunteers, of guinea pigs like himself, persuaded by disposition and circumstance to lend support.

The affliction besets as few as 3 out of every 100,000, although estimates range from this 6,000 in the United States to as many as 50,000 in our population of nearly 210 million.

The problem is not new. Myasthenia gravis is no johnny-come-lately. An Oxonian doctor named Thomas Willis, teaching at Christ Church, described the disorder three hundred years ago. But it was not until 1934 that the most dramatic discovery had been made.

In London, a middle-aged woman found herself unable to carry her shopping bag or prevent her head from falling forward when she knelt to do the hearth. Soon she was bedridden, showing almost all of the classic symptoms of myasthenia gravis.

Lancet, the British medical journal, reported that when Mrs. M was installed in St. Alfrege's Hospital, the senior medical officer, Mary B. Walker, noted that the woman's abnormal muscle fatigue was very much like that induced by curare poison acting on the motor-nerve endings. South American Indians tip their arrows with curare. The alkaloid paralyzes the nervous systems of prey and enemy alike. An antidote had been discovered and Mary Walker tried it on her patient. In her report, she said that "hypodermic injections of physostigmine salisylate acid did have striking, though temporary effect."

When dosages large enough to overcome the muscle weakness were used, the untoward sympathetic explosion was so great that the good effects were smothered in the secondary reactions.

In 1934, on June 16, a new analogue of the curare antidote was developed. Neostigmine methasulphate, called Prostigmine today, inhibits the action of cholinesterase, the chemical that destroys acetylcholine, which is so essential to normal nerve-muscle communications.

Mary Walker began hypodermic injections of "1/60 gram physostigmine sulphate once daily." In thirty minutes to an hour after the injection, the patient's left eyelid went up, arm movement was stronger, the jaw drooped less, swallowing improved, and Mrs. M said she felt "less heavy."

When 1/50 gram of the drug was injected, improvement increased and lasted four to five hours. Still greater improvement resulted from 1/45-gram injections and lasted seven hours. But at this point the patient complained of feeling "rather weak and trembly." Her "insides seemed all on the work" and she felt as if "something be going to happen."

When she was given 1/60 gram by mouth, no detectable effect resulted. However, after 1/30 gram had been administered orally, there was a slight uplift in about an hour. No improvement followed control injections of water, pilocarpine (1/20 gram), strychnine (1/30 gram), adrenalin (5 minims), ephedrine (1/2 gram), and acetylcholine (5/100 and 1/10 gram).

Through the good offices of her counselor and associate, Dr. Philip Hamill, Mary Walker's dramatic case was presented to the Royal Society of Medicine in February of 1935. This attention produced some funds for patient care and increased research, especially in the work of two scientists, Dale and Goddum, who were studying acetylcholine.

Many have worked on the enormous complexities of neuromuscular problems, but no matter how far and deep the research, it will all stem back to that spring day in 1934 when Mary Walker overtook her intuition and applied the deed to it.

To the cast of actors in the intense search for a final answer to this cursed affliction must be added the unfortunate sufferers who have not been improved to recovery by any known therapy. There are some from whom much of value has been learned but upon whom myasthenia gravis has laid so heavy a hand that none of the experts' best efforts have been able to lift it off.

One such was the woman who had been next-door neighbor

to the recovered myasthenic when they both were under treatment at the Clinical Center in Bethesda. Now she was undergoing yet another ACTH course in the ICU ward at Mt. Sinai in Manhattan.

A one-time resident of that room calling to visit her, he donned the slightly grubby medic frock, pushed open the swinging doors, and walked to her bed. Her harassed body was pillow-propped as it had been in countless beds for the past seven years. The mechanical respirator was steadily pumping life into her lungs. Her face was swollen, lips flaked with scraps of skin. She was utterly miserable, torn between wanting to see him and not wanting to be seen.

She was chained by ravaged muscles. Impotent. Almost vegetable—that harrowing state. Unable to exorcise the devils that assailed her. And she was still a young woman, with a sharp mind honed by her malady.

In spite of battle wear, or because of it, there was a dominant demand about her, distressing the nurses who read it as almost a will to failure. She was an impatient patient with, paradoxically, great patience at her command. Her physical strength was formidable in spite of her body weakness, else by now surely she would have succumbed to the beating on that small frame.

This woman had suffered more than two dozen courses of ACTH therapy, many of them back-to-back. She had ingested all manner of drugs and chemicals and had gone through cold turkey withdrawals again and again. Both single- and multi-dose prednisone therapy, which had been the Connecticut myasthenic's salvation, had sent her deep into the well. Never the brass ring. Always the merry-go-round.

Her husband was an enduring and unselfish man, deeply devoted to his wife and their three handsome children, who were growing accustomed to "mother is ill." He was well aware of her nagging concern. How could she manage the children or make a home or be a wife? She did well to stay alive.

There in ICU, as her visitor stood beside her bed, he said what he hoped might tuck even a tinge of hope into a corner of her mind.

"I'm feeling disgustingly fit. If I can do it, anybody can do it."

She looked up at him for a moment. He read the mood at once, knew how she felt, even before she laboriously traced her fingernail across the surface of the child's synthetic slate.

The shaky letters spelled "Not me."

She looked up at him again, then down to the words on the slate. Fumbling, and he knew better than to try to help her, she pulled up the glassine sheet and blotted out the admission of defeat.

At an earlier time, when she had not been laid so low, hers had been an orderly, controlled hand, in keeping with her character. At least it was something to have strength in the fingers when there was none in the chest. She could write in those days even if she couldn't speak. And not in the ill-formed letters she had just erased, which made her doubly angry through frustration.

Prognosis? Weak and unsure. The many consultations had long since confused her as they had her husband. So many therapies had been tried, yet none could go untried. They were straw-grabbers.

As he held her hand and smiled down at her, the visitor recalled his last meeting with her husband. He'd asked how his wife was getting along.

"Not so good. She didn't respond very well to the last ACTH. We've got to try something else."

He was thinking of taking her to Chicago, he'd said, where there was a doctor who'd had favorable reports on the new therapy he was experimenting with. But getting out to the Midwest meant ambulance to airport, ambulance airplane, ambulance to doctor—and back again. With a nurse and an artificial respirator every inch of the way. How do you look after a family and manage a business and try to bring your wife back to life—all at the same time?

"What I understand this doctor does," the husband explained, "is he gives injections of cadicol or whatever it is, and follows it with a hormone builder. Might work. Might not. We just have to try it. It'll cost my right eye."

He paused for a moment, grinned sickly. "So what else is new?"

It has been repeatedly said that no two myasthenics are alike. Here was this woman he had come to visit who had been hammered on like a tribal telegraph. Her lack of adequate responses to any therapy confounded the experts. And there stood her visitor, twice her age, hale and robust from the very drug that had failed her so miserably. Justice is a sometime thing.

After a while he leaned over and kissed the moist forehead

and took his leave. He hadn't told her to hang in there. He didn't have to. He very much hoped there'd be an answer to her burden very soon. And he hoped that until it had been found she wouldn't open her fingers. You will never fall from the cliff if you refuse to open your fingers.

CHAPTER 26

~§ *I am in a moment of prettywellness.*—Horace Walpole

HISTORY rides a carousel.

Lightning does strike twice.

The man who had mastered myasthenia flew back to London in September of 1972. He was met at Heathrow by an old and treasured friend and couldn't resist showing off by lugging the heaviest case out to the Vauxhall.

The Surrey weekend was a feast. English weather at its best. Long walks in the woods. The friendliness of country pubs. And the special pleasure of that charming, sturdy British family.

On the Monday he trained up to London from Claygate, checked into the Savile Club, and basked in the warm staff welcomes. The Savile had been a special club for him ever since he'd heard of the member who wanted to play a rubber or two of bridge one afternoon. Only two tables in the cardroom were occupied. At one they were playing bridge; at the other a somber member was dealing solitaire. After watching the bridge game for a while, the member walked over and knocked into the solitaire game.

The American visitor spent the next day on telephone calls, filling up his calendar and walking in Hyde Park. The Wednesday luncheon with the head of the merchant bank turned out exceptionally well. He took his worn brown shoes to Lobbs for repair, booked several shows (*London Assurance* and *Cowardly*

Custard were particular delights), and made two trips to the British Museum to see the clocks and Scottish holographs.

He walked as if he'd never have another chance to use his legs.

But all this was pale fare to his meeting with Dr. Raymond Greene, who had treated him when he fell apart in London that April thirty months before.

"You cannot know how glad I am to see you looking so well," the tall physician said, smiling broadly as his once-failing patient oversqueezed his hand in greeting. "You have not only made my day, you have made my month."

Over iceless Scotch they probed details of his prednisone therapy, exchanged the names of several moderately priced Parisian restaurants, talked theater, and enjoyed.

The taste of freedom was sweet in the visitor's mouth. There was so much to savor in London, and he constantly overfilled his plate. The drinks at the Garrick Club bar, chuck-elbow with peers of the realm and famous actors. Ribald snooker games—a contradiction in terms—at his own club. Good fellowship in the subterranean Green Room in Adam Street. Game-and-kidney pie, in Samuel Johnson's very own seat, at the Cheshire Cheese, off Fleet Street. He wondered if the illustrious and formidable doctor had ever been called Sammy.

And there was the tasting of the Scotch eggs at the Barley Mow, in Duke Street, with its impressive display of harness brass and the elaborately decorated notice on the inward wall of the alcove.

> Your hands may be dirty
> We don't care two hoots
> But we'd be obliged
> If you'd just wipe your boots

There's a pub in London for every taste. The man who had broken the back of myasthenia had his favorites. He'd always found a specially friendly atmosphere on Tuesdays and Wednesdays, not there the shank of the week, at the thank-you-sir lunches in the Running Footman's upstairs room. And a lusty, noisy, come-one-come-all marked the Seven Stars, in Carey Street off Chancery Lane, where sliced tongue and ale tasted better than they sounded. Particularly when he could share it with the very pretty daughter of his very best friend.

There were several visits to the London Press Club, in Salisbury Square, squired by the talented and eupeptic Eric Williams. Which are adventures not to be sold even a little bit short.

On the eve of his flight to France, he provoked passing smiles by tipping his hat to the notice on the lamppost outside the Savile Club door.

"Litter offenders liable to £100 fine. A person in charge of a dog which fouls the footway is liable to a fine of £20."

They mean it, too. Are you listening, Manhattan?

At Orly he climbed into a Simca and headed south to Chissay-en-Touraine, in the Loire, to visit old friends. Within the week he had re-explored Chenonceau, the most beautiful château in France, and had walked the placid Cher for several kilometers, running memories over in his mind as a miser counts his coins. He and the Gabriel Breuzins went early one morning to Saumur for a special introduction to the fine horses of L'École Grande Cavalerie, and to sample the vintner's private hoard in the cliff-caves of Dampierre-sur-Loire. Roger Pinot's Saumur-Chavigny was ambrosial.

Came adieu time, as it always does. Into the Simca and south to the Dordogne. At a sheltered spot off the road, near Loches, he set out the box of fresh strawberries, the pregnant grapes, a croissant he'd pinched from the breakfast tray, a wedge of Tomme de Savoie. He opened the 1969 Chinon. An emperor's banquet!

As he neared Lalinde, a thirteenth-century village washed by the majestic Dordogne, he savored the rolling hills and the verdure that marked the western edge of the Massif Central and is so like southern New England.

At the appointed hours he would pop medication into his mouth, trying to time it with the Simca's need for fuel. At one station, near Sarlat, he fed the little car as much *essence* as it could swallow, and used the men's room. Over the urinal was the plaint: "Prier de ne pas jeter des magots." It wasn't talking to him. He hadn't put a cigarette to lip in fifteen years.

Toward evening he pulled into Lalinde and parked in the courtyard of the *auberge* his friend had recommended. He relaxed on the terrace that overhung the river, sipped a glass of fine Bordeaux, and watched the patient fishermen on the far side of river contend with gnats and few strikes.

He was up early the next morning, bent on visiting his ancestors. It was a ground-fog morning. What they called tule fog in California. He loafed along the winding roads that led north and west to Les Eyzies, where the Beune and the Vézère meet to form an ideal place for settlement. The rugged scarp of yellow sandstone had presented prehistoric man with a fortress; there, as at Lascaux, a few kilometers north, he had made the caves his home and left his marks upon their walls.

The Connecticut tourist had not come any too soon to view the bones of his forebears. There was talk that the government planned to close the ancient grottos at Les Eyzies as they had at Lascaux. Emanations from the bodies of the visitors, they said, were destructive to the precious wall paintings.

So he gave the guide a few francs, bade farewell to the old folks at home, and easy-rode in perfect weather toward Paris. When he arrived, having turned in the Simca at Orly, there were meetings with friends, favorite restaurants were revisited, and he took long and rewarding walks. And the point of it all was that he was doing it all on his own.

Homeward bound now. The purring VC-10 was slower and smaller than the flying barns. And no movies. He liked it better. Sat back and relaxed. The French pilgrimage was history now and he'd seen his beloved London once again, walking the streets that had been torment to him two short years before with strong and even stride, charging his lungs with the sweetest of all wines.

Sir Andrew Barton had said it well, a hundred years before the Plague and the Great Fire, on a battlefield not far from London:

> Fight on, my men, and press the foe.
> A little I'm hurt but not yet slain.
> I will lie me here and bleed a while
> And then I'll rise and fight again.

APPENDICES

APPENDIX 1

When found, make a note of it.—Dombey and Son

Throughout the Connecticut myasthenic's illness, he kept a daily record of his responses to treatment, if he was able to do so. The following entries cover six weeks in 1970, prior to his admission to the National Institute of Neurological Diseases and Stroke, Bethesda, Maryland.

Jan. 1 —Bkfst swallow adequate but better last wk. Dr: "Go up 1 cc. Mestinon at 6 A.M. to 2 cc."

Jan. 2 —Nuthin! Lousy.

Jan. 3 —Swallow off badly. Unless it is liquid, food hangs on shelf at back of throat. Wgt down to 150. Slightest exertion gives fatigue. Am ten days out of (Greenwich) hospital. Think I should be stronger by now. Dinner bad tonight. Swallowing very difficult.

Jan. 4 —Same as ystdy. Slight diplopia in early A.M.

Jan. 5 —Dr: "Start new time cycle: 1½ cc. Mestinon (18 mg.) at 7 A.M., 12 noon, 5 P.M., 10 P.M." Speech slurred abruptly in middle of lunch. Nuts. Lips weak. Breath short. Speech very slurred by 5 P.M. Can't swallow anything but liquids. They're no fun, either.

Jan. 6 —Swallowing same as ystdy. Legs weaker.

Jan. 7 —Swallow better today but not much. Dr: "Go down 6 mg. at 7 A.M. Experiment for two–three days. Check effect." Let him know. Have to go slow on ACTH shots. Gotta have Bird (respirator) handy in case chest muscles poop out. Had a bad night. Up a dozen times.

Jan. 8 —Down to 1 cc. at 7 A.M. Swallow/lips/speech NG. Chewing way off at dinner. Dysphagia (swallowing difficulty) pronounced. Went up to 2 cc. Mestinon at 6 P.M.

Jan. 9 —More of same. Sheesh.

Jan. 10—Put in new trach-tube. Metal. Stoma uncomfortable. Smells infected.

Jan. 11—Tensilon test at clinic. Dr: "Go up a little on each dose." Fixed up stoma infection. Bkfst/Lunch/Dinner NG despite 2½ cc.

Jan. 12—Same. Stoma bothers. Air leakage. Bad chewing. Food hangs on shelf. Hard to dislodge.

Jan. 13—Forget it.

Jan. 14—Chewing/swallowing/speech definitely going downhill.

Jan. 15—Swallowing out! Poured milk to wash Mestinon down. Eyes weak *and* diplopia. Caught cold. Sneezing. Bad day overall.

Jan. 16—Weight 148. Symptoms about same. Dr. says new technique developed involving destruction of bad lymphocytes which seem to be immobilized by ACTH but not killed. Injection of antilymphocyte serum (from cows, horses) difficult to get. Side effects: cancer, red cell destruction. Told Dr. they could try it on me. Nothing else doing much good.

Jan. 17—More of same. Dismal day.

Jan. 18—Woke after bloody dreams. Bad sleep. Symptoms up all day.

Jan. 19—Dr. O (Kermit Osserman): "Mytelase no good to activate throat muscles. Mestinon won't either. Weekly ACTH best method we've found. When it works. Must have Bird or Bennett (respirators) and suction-machine on hand. Some patients shot on Fri, weaken by Sun, revive Mon or Tues." Sounds awful guessy, unpredictable but ain't sitting in choosy seat.

Jan. 20—Bad day. All three meals NG.

Jan. 21—Dinner NG. Barely got pap food washed down. More gravity than swallowing.

Jan. 22—Same. Went up to 2 cc. Mestinon 5 P.M. & 10 P.M.

Jan. 23—Much mucus. Breathing restricted. Very bad dysphagia.

178

Chewing off again. Took 3 cc. at 5 P.M. Put in new #6 silver trach-tube. Stoma very uncomfortable.

Jan. 24—Chew/swall weaker. Throat sore as hell.

Jan. 25—Chewing weaker by lunch. Don't want to try for food. Speech NG. Feel lousy.

Jan. 26—Stoma hurts quite badly now. Dr. says try #7 trach-tube. Too big. Cut flesh. Little bleeding. Much mucus. All symptoms yoyo.

Jan. 27—"Let's give it another day." Shit. Gave.

Jan. 28—Dr. C gave ACTH injection. 3 P.M. 100 units. No change by midnight. Not bad sleep.

Jan. 29—Clinic. Tensilon showed "underdosed." Up ½ cc.

Jan. 30—Bad day. All bulbar symptoms stink. Heavy ptosis at noon. 2 P.M. to (Greenwich Hospital) clinic. Tensilon: "underdosed." Dr. fearful of overdosing. Set Mestinon at 3 cc. for 5 P.M. and 10 P.M. We ain't getting nowhere fast in leaky handbasket.

Jan. 31—7 A.M. Swallowing improved! Can't figger it. 10 A.M.: both eyes weak; much ptosis. Swallowing went off at 1 P.M. No chewing now. Barely got Mestinon down. Slow pour for gravity. No lunch but hungry. 2 P.M. to clinic. Positive response to Tensilon. 5 P.M.: 4 cc. 10 P.M.: 3 cc.

Feb. 1 —Swallow fair at 7 A.M. Lip/chewing fatigue rapidly at 9. Recovery slower than ever before. Ptosis bad. Speech slurring again. No lunch. To hell with it. To clinic at 1 P.M. Tensilon: "underdosed." Back to 4 cc. at 5 P.M. Dinner NG *in toto*. Can barely flow medicine down with milk.

Feb. 2 —4 cc. at 7 A.M. Bkfst—ehh. Swallow up a little at 9 A.M. Speech fatigues quickly. Ptosis heavy. Dr. C: "Take 3 cc. at 10 P.M. If feel okay next morn, take 1 cc." Sounds dumb but he ought to know. Dinner out the window. Dumb evening.

Feb. 3 —Dysphagia same as ystdy. Clinic. Tensilon: "underdosed." Back up to 4 cc. Mestinon at noon. Swallow worst in days. Just ain't there at all. Took 5½ cc. at 5 P.M. Dinner NG at all. Chew gone with swallow. First time in long time neck muscles weaker. Took 4½ cc. at 10 P.M. Had to wash it down. Don't think am taking enough. Slight aspiration. Much coughing. Feel won't be able to wash down safely much longer.

Feb. 4 —All meals NG. Not much change from ystdy. Took 6½ cc. at 6 P.M. No reaction.

Feb. 5 —Very bad headache at 6 A.M. Took 6½ cc. Mestinon at 7. No chew at bkfst but slight swallow!?! Up to 8 cc. (96 mg.) at 5 P.M.

Feb. 6 —Took 8 cc. at 7 and noon. Throat seems to be closing. Get weaker all over as day progresses. Very short of breath after few words. Slurred. Took 9 cc. at 5 P.M. and 10 P.M. Neck muscles weaker. Very bad night.

Feb. 7 —7 A.M. took 9½ cc. Mestinon. Took 10 cc. at noon. Very short of breath by 4 P.M., even with no exertion. 10 cc. at 5 P.M. and 10 P.M. Nothing happened.

Feb. 8 —Took 10 cc. at 7, 12, 5, 10 P.M. Much worse. Think I'm losing.

Feb. 9 —Going downhill fast. Breathing very difficult. Dr. insists I go to hospital. So go.

Feb. 10—Feel like hell. All symptoms no bloody go.

Feb. 11—Up to 11 cc. 4td (four times daily). No help.

Feb. 12—Up to 12 cc. 5td! NG.

Feb. 13—12 cc 5td. No change.

Feb. 14—Now up to 12½ cc. 5td. Be my valentine. Worst yet.

Feb. 15—More of same only lousier. Breathing definitely leaving town. Better get help soon or else.

By noon on February 15, 1970, the myasthenic went onto artificial respiration. A nasogastric tube was inserted for food and medication.

APPENDIX 2

In the NEW ENGLAND JOURNAL OF MEDICINE, January 6, 1972, Dr. W. King Engel and Dr. John R. Warmolts, of the Medical Neurology Branch of National Institute of Neurological Diseases and Stroke, Bethesda, Maryland, made the following observations and case-history report:

The ordinary myasthenia gravis therapy with cholinesterase inhibitors at frequent, precisely-spaced intervals during the day provides improvement that lasts only a few hours, is usually incomplete and may greatly diminish after some months' duration.

In some patients, favorable longer-term results may follow thymectomy, short-term courses of massive amounts of ACTH, or longer-term periodic ACTH injections.

In five consecutive case-studies of adults with myasthenia gravis, lasting improvement was achieved through the use of long-term, high (100 mg), single-dosage, alternate-day oral prednisone therapy.

Prednisone was given in single morning dose, without anticholinesterase medication, supplemented by 15 to 30 mEq of potassium ion four times a day, antacids through each day, low sodium and carbohydrate diet, and elaborate respiratory and nursing attendance during the early phases of the treatment.

[They say this about the Connecticut patient:]

A 68-year-old man had a 2½-year history of generalized myasthenia, improved by anticholinesterase drugs but not by thymectomy. Four subsequent ACTH courses (short-term) for continuing deterioration each led to three weeks temporary improvement, after a period of worsening during ACTH administration, although anticholinesterases were concomitantly increased.

For a year before admission (to NIH) a permanent tracheostomy orifice was maintained. Continuing deterioration led to inability to swallow in one month and need for nearly continuous respiration two weeks after admission.

Effective withdrawl of the 125mg of pyridostigmine bromide, taken every four hours, further increased the marked bulbar and moderate limb weakness found on admission. Ulnar nerve stimulation at 1, 2, 5, 10, and 20 per second invoked a prominent decrementing response from abductor digiti quinti.

Detectable subtle improvement, beginning with the second dose of alternate-day prednisone therapy, appeared first in the fore-arms and then arms, respiratory, tongue, and, finally, facial muscles. During the early on-prednisone days, improved strength and endurance could be detected clinically in two to four hours, reached a maximum in ten to 12 hours, then subsided to an overall improved level of strength until further benefit followed the next prednisone dose.

The patient responded to prednisone at the second dose (fourth day). There were repeated upsurge and fall-off (though not to or below previous levels) during the first three weeks.

By the 17th day of treatment, strength and endurance on prednisone surpassed that of admission to NIH, when the patient was receiving cholinesterase inhibitors. By four weeks into the therapy, the respirator was no longer required, and he was active on the ward. However, after eight weeks improvement he reached a plateau, with nasogastric feeding and frequent rest periods required.

After three weeks into continued therapy, mild fore-arm and neck erector muscle weakness reappeared. An increase in prednisone to 175mg alternating with 50mg as single doses on successive mornings was followed by return of fore-arm and neck strength, improvement in general endurance and, six months into therapy, by swallowing adequate for nutrition.

With subsequent reduction of prednisone to 175mg on alternate mornings only, improvement had been maintained. The patient now travels freely by public airplane.

APPENDIX 3

There is an extensive library on myasthenia gravis. Thomas Willis is credited with the first clinical description of myasthenia gravis in "Two Discourses Concerning the Soul of Brutes," published in London in 1683. Detailed reports were made in the nineteenth century by Drs. Erb and Goldflam, by whose names the malady was known for many years. Sir Samuel Wilks, a physician to Guy's Hospital in London, presented a detailed account in 1877. It was in 1895 that a German doctor, F. Jolly, became the first to apply the name "myasthenia gravis pseudo-paralytica" to the disease. In 1904 and 1905, Otto Gruner and Johannes Kollner wrote the Kronisberg and Berlin theses on myasthenia, and Louis Boudon published a paper entitled "La Myasthénie Grave, Anatome Pathologique et Pathogénie" in 1909. Twenty years elapsed before another Frenchman, Pierre Bourgoise, delivered his "Contribution à l'Etude de la Myasthénie."

The Myasthenia Gravis Foundation, 12 East 103rd Street, New York, New York 10029, can supply a fund of contemporary information on myasthenia gravis. The following references are available:

Engel, W. King, and Warmolts, John R. "Benefit from Alternate-Day Prednisone in Myasthenia Gravis." *New England Journal of Medicine*, Vol. 286 (1972), pp. 17–20.
——. "Myasthenia Gravis—A New Hypothesis of the Pathogenesis and a New Form of Treatment." *Annals of the New York Academy of Sciences*, Vol. 183 (1971), pp. 72–87.

Fields, W. S. "Myasthenia Gravis." *Annals of the New York Academy of Sciences*, Vol. 183 (1971).

Merritt, Houston. *Textbook on Neurology*. Philadelphia: Lea & Febiger, 1967.

Osserman, Kermit E., editor, "Myasthenia Gravis." *Annals of the New York Academy of Sciences*, Vol. 135 (1966).

Osserman, Kermit E., and Strauss, A. J. L., "Myasthenia Gravis," *Immunological Diseases*, edited by M. Samter and H. L. Alexander. Boston: Little, Brown & Co., 1965.

Osserman, Kermit E., and Genkins, Gabriel. "Myasthenia Gravis—Short-Term Massive Cortico-Tropin (ACTH) Therapy." *Journal of American Medical Association*, Vol. 198 (1966), pp. 699–702.

Patten, Bernard M., Oliver, Katharine L., and Engel, W. King. "Adverse Interaction between Corticosteroid Hormones and Anti-Cholinesterase Drugs." *Transactions of the American Neurological Association*, Vol. 98 (1973).

Viets, Henry R. *Myasthenia Gravis*. Springfield, Ill.: Grune & Stratton, 1961.

Walker, M. B. "Treatment of Myasthenia Gravis with Physiostigmine." *Lancet*, Vol. I (1934), p. 1200.